SIBO BIPHASIC DIET COOKBOOK

Easy and Delicious Gut-Friendly Recipes

Peggy C. Valentine

COPYRIGHTS

© [2024] by **Peggy C. Valentine**

TABLE OF CONTENTS

Chapter 1:

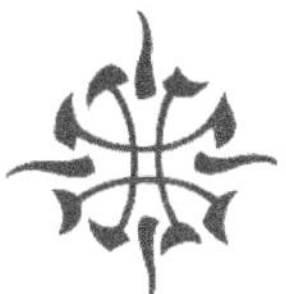

INTRODUCTION TO THE SIBO BIPHASIC DIET

1. SIBO, which stands for Small Intestinal Bacterial Overgrowth, is a digestive disorder characterized by an excessive growth of bacteria in the small intestine. Normally, the small intestine has a relatively low bacterial count compared to the large intestine. However, in SIBO, bacteria from the large intestine migrate and multiply in the small intestine, leading to various symptoms and complications.

When it comes to the diet and SIBO, it's essential to understand that different types of carbohydrates can exacerbate the condition. Bacteria in the small intestine ferment undigested carbohydrates, producing gases and causing symptoms like bloating, abdominal pain, diarrhea, and constipation. Therefore, managing your diet is crucial in reducing symptoms and promoting gut healing.

The SIBO diet typically focuses on reducing or eliminating certain types of carbohydrates that are known to ferment easily. This includes avoiding high-FODMAP foods, which stands for Fermentable Oligosaccharides, Disaccharides, Monosaccharides, and Polyols. These carbohydrates are poorly absorbed in the small intestine and can fuel bacterial overgrowth, leading to symptoms.

The SIBO diet often involves limiting or avoiding foods such as onions, garlic, wheat, rye, legumes, certain fruits, dairy products, and sweeteners like sorbitol and xylitol. Instead, it emphasizes consuming easily digestible and low-FODMAP foods such as lean proteins, non-starchy vegetables, some fruits, gluten-free grains, and healthy fats.

It's important to note that the SIBO diet is not a one-size-fits-all approach. The severity of your symptoms, specific bacterial strains involved, and individual tolerances may vary. Therefore, working with a healthcare professional or a registered dietitian experienced in SIBO is highly recommended to tailor the diet to your unique needs.

2. The Biphasic approach in SIBO treatment involves two distinct phases: Phase 1 and Phase 2. Understanding these phases is essential for effectively managing SIBO and promoting gut healing.

Phase 1 is the Restrictive Phase, also known as the Elimination Phase. During this phase, the primary goal is to starve the overgrown bacteria by following a strict diet that limits fermentable carbohydrates. The duration of Phase 1 typically ranges from two to four weeks, depending on the individual's response and severity of symptoms.

In Phase 1, you will eliminate high-FODMAP foods, which are known to worsen SIBO symptoms. This helps to reduce bacterial fermentation and alleviate digestive distress. The diet during this phase mainly consists of easily digestible proteins, low-FODMAP vegetables, some fruits, gluten-free grains, and healthy fats. It's important to strictly adhere to the recommended food list and portion sizes to achieve optimal results.

After completing Phase 1, you will transition to Phase 2, which is the Reintroduction Phase. This phase focuses on gradually reintroducing specific carbohydrates to determine your individual tolerance levels. By reintroducing one type of carbohydrate at a time, you can identify which foods trigger symptoms and which ones can be safely included in your diet.

The duration of Phase 2 varies depending on your response to different carbohydrates. It's crucial to keep a food and symptom diary during this phase to track your reactions to specific foods. This information will help guide your dietary choices and create a personalized long-term eating plan.

The Biphasic approach aims to not only address the immediate symptoms of SIBO but also identify the root causes and provide long-term management strategies. By following both Phase 1 and Phase 2, you can effectively manage your diet to alleviate symptoms, promote gut healing, and maintain a healthy balance of gut bacteria.

3. Implementing the SIBO Biphasic diet successfully requires careful planning and preparation. Here are some tips to help you navigate the process and maximize your chances of achieving positive outcomes:

a. Educate Yourself: Take the time to understand the basics of SIBO, its symptoms, and how the Biphasic diet can help. Familiarize yourself with the recommended foods and those to avoid during each phase. Resources such as books, reputable websites, and guidance from healthcare professionals can provide valuable information.

b. Consult a Healthcare Professional: Work with a knowledgeable healthcare professional, preferably one experienced in SIBO and nutrition, to guide you through the diet implementation process. They can assess your specific needs, provide personalized recommendations, and monitor your progress.

c. Plan your Meals: Meal planning is crucial to ensure you have suitable options available throughout the day. Create a meal plan for each phase, incorporating a variety of low-FODMAP foods that you enjoy. This will make grocery shopping and meal preparation more manageable.

d. Stock SIBO-Friendly Foods: Prioritize stocking your pantry and refrigerator with SIBO-friendly ingredients. This includes lean proteins like chicken, turkey, and fish, low-FODMAP vegetables, gluten-free grains, healthy fats, and suitable condiments and seasonings. Having these items readily available will help you stickto your diet and avoid temptation or frustration.

e. Prepare in Advance: Dedicate time to meal preparation and batch cooking. This will save you time and effort during busy days when you may be tempted to choose convenient but unsuitable foods. Prepare meals and snacks in advance, portion them out, and store them for easy access throughout the week.

f. Stay Hydrated: Adequate hydration is essential for overall health and digestion. Drink plenty of water throughout the day to support proper gut function and promote regular bowel movements. Hydration also helps to prevent constipation, a common issue in SIBO.

g. Seek Support: Living with SIBO and following a restricted diet can be challenging. Reach out to support groups, online communities, or friends and family who can provide encouragement, understanding, and helpful tips. Sharing experiences and learning from others can make the journey more manageable.

h. Monitor and Adjust: Keep track of your symptoms, food reintroductions, and any changes in your condition. This will help you identify patterns, trigger foods, and necessary adjustments to your diet. Regularly communicate with your healthcare professional to discuss your progress and make any necessary modifications.

Remember, the successful implementation of the SIBO Biphasic diet requires patience, perseverance, and a commitment to your health. Stay focused on your goals, listen to your body, and seek professional guidance when needed. With time, effort, and the right approach, you can find relief from SIBO symptoms and improve your overall well-being.

4. The SIBO Biphasic diet can be made more manageable and effective with the right tools and ingredients in your kitchen. Here are some essential items to consider:

a. Kitchen Tools:

- Cutting Board and Knife: A sturdy cutting board and sharp knife are essential for prepping vegetables, fruits, and proteins.

- Cookware: Invest in a variety of cookware, including pots, pans, and baking sheets, to accommodate different cooking methods. Non-stick options can be helpful for minimizing the use of added fats.

- Kitchen Scale: A kitchen scale allows you to measure ingredients precisely, which is important when following portion sizes and specific recipes.

- Blender or Food Processor: These appliances can be useful for creating sauces, purees, or blending smoothies using approved ingredients.

- Steamer Basket: Steaming vegetables is a gentle cooking method that helps retain nutrients while making them easier to digest.

- Slow Cooker or Instant Pot: These versatile appliances can simplify meal preparation, especially when you're short on time. They allow for hands-off cooking and are ideal for preparing stews, soups, and tender meats.

b. Essential Ingredients:

- Lean Proteins: Stock up on lean protein sources such as chicken, turkey, fish, and eggs. These can be cooked in various ways to add variety to your meals.

- Low-FODMAP Vegetables: Include a range of low-FODMAP vegetables like spinach, kale, zucchini, bell peppers, carrots, and cucumbers. These provide essential nutrients while being gentle on the digestive system.

- Gluten-Free Grains: Opt for gluten-free grains like quinoa, rice, millet, and buckwheat as a source of carbohydrates. These grains are less likely to trigger symptoms.

- Healthy Fats: Choose healthy fats such as olive oil, coconut oil, avocado oil, and ghee. These can be used for cooking, dressings, or added to meals for flavor and satiety.

- Herbs and Spices: Enhance the taste of your dishes with a variety of herbs and spices like basil, oregano, turmeric, ginger, cumin, and cinnamon. They can add depth and complexity to your meals without adding FODMAPs.

- Low-FODMAP Fruits: Select low-FODMAP fruits such as berries, citrus fruits, and melons for added sweetness. These can be enjoyed in moderation during Phase 2.

By having these essential kitchen tools and ingredients on hand, you'll be well-prepared to create delicious and compliant meals throughout your SIBO Biphasic diet journey.

5. Making modifications and substitutions in recipes while following the SIBO Biphasic diet is crucial to accommodate your dietary restrictions and preferences. Here are some key principles to keep in mind:

a. Replace High-FODMAP Ingredients: Identify high-FODMAP ingredients in recipes and find suitable replacements. For example, substitute onions and garlic with garlic-infused oil or use herbs like chives or scallions (green parts only) for flavor.

b. Adjust Sweeteners: Many recipes call for high-FODMAP sweeteners like honey, agave syrup, or high-fructose corn syrup. Instead, opt for low-FODMAP sweeteners such as maple syrup, stevia, or small amounts of cane sugar.

c. Choose Gluten-Free Alternatives: If a recipe includes gluten-containing ingredients like wheat flour, choose gluten-free alternatives such as rice flour, almond flour, or gluten-free baking mixes.

Chapter 2:

BREAKFAST DELIGHTS

Scrambled Eggs with Green Veggies:

- Preparation time: 10 minutes

- Cooking time: 10 minutes

- Servings: 2

Ingredients:

- 4 large eggs

- 1 cup chopped spinach

- 1/2 cup diced zucchini

- 1/2 cup diced bell peppers

- 2 tablespoons olive oil

- Salt and pepper to taste

Directions:

1. In a bowl, whisk the eggs until well beaten. Set aside.

2. Heat olive oil in a non-stick skillet over medium heat.

3. Add the chopped spinach, diced zucchini, and diced bell peppers to the skillet. Sauté for about 3-4 minutes until the vegetables are tender.

4. Pour the beaten eggs into the skillet and gently scramble them with the vegetables until cooked to your desired consistency.

5. Season with salt and pepper to taste.

6. Serve the scrambled eggs with green veggies hot and enjoy!

Nutritional Information (per serving):

- Calories: 225

- Protein: 14g

- Fat: 16g

- Carbohydrates: 6g

- Fiber: 2g

Quinoa Breakfast Bowl:

- Preparation time: 5 minutes

- Cooking time: 15 minutes

- Servings: 2

Ingredients:

- 1 cup cooked quinoa

- 1/2 cup unsweetened almond milk

- 1/2 cup mixed berries (e.g., strawberries, blueberries, raspberries)

- 2 tablespoons chopped nuts (e.g., almonds, walnuts)

- 1 tablespoon unsweetened shredded coconut

- 1 teaspoon honey or maple syrup (optional)

Directions:

1. In a saucepan, heat the cooked quinoa and almond milk over medium heat until warmed through.

2. Divide the quinoa mixture into two bowls.

3. Top each bowl with mixed berries, chopped nuts, and shredded coconut.

4. Drizzle with honey or maple syrup if desired.

5. Serve the quinoa breakfast bowl warm and enjoy!

Nutritional Information (per serving):

- Calories: 235

- Protein: 8g

- Fat: 10g

- Carbohydrates: 30g

- Fiber: 8g

Almond Flour Pancakes:

- Preparation time: 10 minutes

- Cooking time: 10 minutes

- Servings: 2-3 (approximately 6 small pancakes)

Ingredients:

- 1 cup almond flour

- 2 large eggs

- 1/4 cup unsweetened almond milk

- 1 tablespoon coconut oil (melted)

- 1 tablespoon maple syrup (optional)

- 1/2 teaspoon baking powder

- 1/2 teaspoon vanilla extract

- Pinch of salt

Directions:

1. In a bowl, whisk together the almond flour, eggs, almond milk, coconut oil, maple syrup (if using), baking powder, vanilla extract, and salt until well combined.

2. Heat a non-stick skillet or griddle over medium heat.

3. Scoop about 1/4 cup of the batter onto the skillet for each pancake.

4. Cook until bubbles form on the surface, then flip and cook for another 1-2 minutes until golden brown.

5. Repeat with the remaining batter.

6. Serve the almond flour pancakes hot with your favorite SIBO-friendly toppings such as fresh berries or a dollop of almond butter.

Nutritional Information (per serving, based on 3 servings):

- Calories: 268

- Protein: 11g

- Fat: 22g

- Carbohydrates: 8g

- Fiber: 4g

Avocado Toast with Poached Eggs:

- Preparation time: 10 minutes

- Cooking time: 5 minutes

- Servings: 2

Ingredients:

- 2 slices of gluten-free bread (toasted)

- 1 ripe avocado (pitted and mashed)

- 2 large eggs (poached)

- Salt and pepper to taste

- Optional toppings: sliced cherry tomatoes, fresh herbs (e.g., cilantro, basil)

Directions:

1. Toast the slices of gluten-free bread until golden brown.

2. Spread the mashed avocado evenly on each slice of toast.

3. Top each slice with a poached egg.

4. Season with salt and pepper to taste.

5. Add optional toppings like sliced cherry tomatoes or fresh herbs.

6. Serve the avocado toast with poached eggs immediately.

Nutritional Information (per serving):

- Calories: 285

- Protein: 13g

- Fat: 20g

- Carbohydrates: 14g

- Fiber: 8g

Spinach and Feta Omelette:

- Preparation time: 10 minutes

- Cooking time: 10 minutes

- Servings: 1

Ingredients:

- 2 large eggs

- 1/2 cup fresh spinach leaves

- 1/4 cup crumbled feta cheese

- 1 tablespoon olive oil

- Salt and pepper to taste

Directions:

1. In a bowl, whisk the eggs until well beaten. Set aside.

2. Heat olive oil in a non-stick skillet over medium heat.

3. Add the fresh spinach leaves to the skillet and sauté for about 2 minutes until wilted.

4. Pour the beaten eggs into the skillet, tilting the pan to spread the eggs evenly.

5. Cook for a few minutes until the edges start to set.

6. Sprinkle the crumbled feta cheese evenly over one half of the omelette.

7. Fold the other half of the omelette over the filling.

8. Cook for another minute until the cheese is melted and the omelette is cooked through.

9. Season with salt and pepper to taste.

10. Serve the spinach and feta omelette hot and enjoy!

Nutritional Information (per serving):

- Calories: 295

- Protein: 22g

- Fat: 21g

- Carbohydrates: 3g

- Fiber: 1g

Chia Pudding with Berries:

- Preparation time: 5 minutes (plus chilling time)

- Cooking time: No cooking required

- Servings: 2

Ingredients:

- 1/4 cup chia seeds

- 1 cup unsweetened almond milk (or any other non-dairy milk)

- 1 tablespoon maple syrup (or sweetener of choice)

- 1/2 teaspoon vanilla extract

- 1/2 cup mixed berries (e.g., strawberries, blueberries, raspberries)

- Optional toppings: chopped nuts, coconut flakes, or additional berries

Directions:

1. In a bowl, whisk together the chia seeds, almond milk, maple syrup, and vanilla extract until well combined.

2. Let the mixture sit for 5 minutes, then whisk again to prevent clumping.

3. Cover the bowl and refrigerate for at least 2 hours or overnight until the chia pudding thickens.

4. Once chilled, give the pudding a good stir to break up any clumps.

5. Divide the chia pudding into serving bowls or jars.

6. Top with mixed berries and any desired toppings.

7. Serve the chia pudding with berries chilled and enjoy!

Nutritional Information (per serving):

- Calories: 160

- Protein: 5g

- Fat: 8g

- Carbohydrates: 17g

- Fiber: 9g

Sweet Potato Hash with Turkey Sausage:

- Preparation time: 15 minutes

- Cooking time: 25 minutes

- Servings: 2

Ingredients:

- 2 small sweet potatoes (peeled and diced)

- 4 ounces turkey sausage (casings removed)

- 1/2 onion (diced)

- 1 bell pepper (diced)

- 1 tablespoon olive oil

- 1 teaspoon dried thyme

- 1/2 teaspoon paprika

- Salt and pepper to taste

- Optional toppings: chopped fresh parsley or green onions

Directions:

1. Heat olive oil in a skillet over medium heat.

2. Add the diced sweet potatoes and cook for about 8-10 minutes until they start to soften.

3. Add the turkey sausage, onion, and bell pepper to the skillet. Cook for another 8-10 minutes until the sausage is cooked through and the vegetables are tender.

4. Add the dried thyme, paprika, salt, and pepper. Stir to combine.

5. Continue cooking for a few more minutes until the flavors meld together.

6. Remove from heat and sprinkle with optional toppings.

7. Serve the sweet potato hash with turkey sausage hot and enjoy!

Nutritional Information (per serving):

- Calories: 285

- Protein: 12g

- Fat: 12g

- Carbohydrates: 36g

- Fiber: 6g

Gluten-Free Banana Bread:

- Preparation time: 15 minutes

- Cooking time: 50-60 minutes

- Servings: 12 slices

Ingredients:

- 2 cups mashed ripe bananas (about 4 medium bananas)

- 4 large eggs

- 1/2 cup coconut flour

- 1/2 cup almond flour

- 1/4 cup coconut oil (melted)

- 1/4 cup honey or maple syrup

- 1 teaspoon vanilla extract

- 1 teaspoon baking soda

- 1/2 teaspoon cinnamon

- Pinch of salt

- Optional add-ins: chopped nuts, chocolate chips

Directions:

1. Preheat the oven to 350°F (175°C). Grease a loaf pan with coconut oil or line it with parchment paper.

2. In a large bowl, whisk together the mashed bananas, eggs, coconut flour, almond flour, coconut oil, honey or maple syrup, vanilla extract, baking soda, cinnamon, and salt until well combined.

3. If desired, stir in optional add-ins like chopped nuts or chocolate chips.

4. Pour the batter into the prepared loaf pan and spread it evenly.

5. Bake for 50-60 minutes, or until a toothpick inserted into the center comes out clean.

6. Allow the banana bread to cool in the pan for 10 minutes, then transfer it to a wire rack to cool completely.

7. Once cooled, slice the gluten-free banana bread into individual servings.

8. Serve the banana bread slices at room temperature and enjoy!

Nutritional Information (per serving, based on 12 slices):

- Calories: 165

- Protein: 4g

- Fat: 9g

- Carbohydrates: 19g

- Fiber: 4g

Greek Yogurt Parfait:

- Preparation time: 5 minutes

- Cooking time: No cooking required

- Servings: 1

Ingredients:

- 1 cup plainGreek yogurt

- 1/2 cup mixed berries (e.g., strawberries, blueberries, raspberries)

- 2 tablespoons granola

- 1 tablespoon honey or maple syrup

- Optional toppings: chopped nuts, coconut flakes, or additional berries

Directions:

1. In a glass or jar, layer half of the Greek yogurt.

2. Add half of the mixed berries on top of the yogurt.

3. Sprinkle 1 tablespoon of granola over the berries.

4. Drizzle 1/2 tablespoon of honey or maple syrup on top.

5. Repeat the layers with the remaining ingredients.

6. Finish with optional toppings like chopped nuts, coconut flakes, or additional berries.

7. Serve the Greek yogurt parfait chilled and enjoy!

Nutritional Information (per serving):

- Calories: 280

- Protein: 23g

- Fat: 6g

- Carbohydrates: 40g

- Fiber: 4g

Zucchini and Carrot Fritters:

- Preparation time: 15 minutes

- Cooking time: 15 minutes

- Servings: 4

Ingredients:

- 2 medium zucchini (grated)

- 2 medium carrots (grated)

- 1/2 onion (finely chopped)

- 1/4 cup gluten-free flour (e.g., rice flour or chickpea flour)

- 2 large eggs (lightly beaten)

- 2 tablespoons chopped fresh parsley

- 1/2 teaspoon baking powder

- Salt and pepper to taste

- Olive oil (for frying)

Directions:

1. Place the grated zucchini and carrots in a clean kitchen towel or cheesecloth. Squeeze out any excess moisture.

2. In a large bowl, combine the grated zucchini, carrots, chopped onion, gluten-free flour, eggs, parsley, baking powder, salt, and pepper. Mix well until all ingredients are evenly incorporated.

3. Heat a thin layer of olive oil in a skillet over medium heat.

4. Spoon about 2 tablespoons of the vegetable mixture onto the skillet, flattening it with the back of the spoon to form a fritter. Repeat with the remaining mixture, leaving some space between each fritter.

5. Cook the fritters for 3-4 minutes per side, or until golden brown and crispy.

6. Once cooked, transfer the fritters to a paper towel-lined plate to absorb any excess oil.

7. Repeat the process with the remaining vegetable mixture.

8. Serve the zucchini and carrot fritters warm as a delicious breakfast option!

Nutritional Information (per serving, about 2 fritters):

- Calories: 150

- Protein: 6g

- Fat: 6g

- Carbohydrates: 19g

- Fiber: 4g

Blueberry Coconut Smoothie Bowl:

- Preparation time: 5 minutes

- Cooking time: No cooking required

- Servings: 1

Ingredients:

- 1 frozen banana

- 1/2 cup frozen blueberries

- 1/2 cup coconut milk (or any other milk of your choice)

- 1 tablespoon almond butter (or any nut butter)

- Toppings: fresh blueberries, shredded coconut, sliced almonds, chia seeds

Directions:

1. In a blender, combine the frozen banana, frozen blueberries, coconut milk, and almond butter.

2. Blend until smooth and creamy.

3. Pour the smoothie into a bowl.

4. Top with fresh blueberries, shredded coconut, sliced almonds, and chia seeds.

5. Serve the blueberry coconut smoothie bowl immediately and enjoy!

Baked Oatmeal with Apples and Cinnamon:

- Preparation time: 10 minutes

- Cooking time: 30 minutes

- Servings: 4

Ingredients:

- 2 cups rolled oats

- 1 teaspoon baking powder

- 1/2 teaspoon ground cinnamon

- 1/4 teaspoon salt

- 1 1/2 cups almond milk (or any other milk of your choice)

- 1/4 cup maple syrup (or sweetener of choice)

- 1 large egg

- 1 teaspoon vanilla extract

- 1 apple (peeled, cored, and chopped)

- Optional toppings: chopped nuts, extra cinnamon, maple syrup

Directions:

1. Preheat the oven to 350°F (175°C). Grease a baking dish with coconut oil or cooking spray.

2. In a large bowl, mix together the rolled oats, baking powder, ground cinnamon, and salt.

3. In a separate bowl, whisk together the almond milk, maple syrup, egg, and vanilla extract.

4. Add the wet ingredients to the dry ingredients and stir until well combined.

5. Stir in the chopped apple.

6. Pour the mixture into the prepared baking dish and spread it evenly.

7. Bake for 30 minutes or until the top is golden brown and the oatmeal is set.

8. Remove from the oven and let it cool for a few minutes.

9. Serve the baked oatmeal with apples and cinnamon warm, and add optional toppings if desired.

Smoked Salmon and Dill Frittata:

Preparation time: 10 minutes

- Cooking time: 20 minutes

- Servings: 4

Ingredients:

- 8 large eggs

- 1/4 cup milk

- 4 ounces smoked salmon, chopped

- 1/4 cup chopped fresh dill

- 1/2 cup chopped red onion

- Salt and pepper to taste

- 1 tablespoon olive oil

Directions:

1. Preheat the oven to 350°F (175°C).

2. In a bowl, whisk together the eggs and milk.

3. Stir in the chopped smoked salmon, fresh dill, red onion, salt, and pepper.

4. Heat olive oil in an oven-safe skillet over medium heat.

5. Pour the egg mixture into the skillet and cook for 2-3 minutes until the edges start to set.

6. Transfer the skillet to the preheated oven and bake for 15-18 minutes or until the frittata is set in the center.

7. Remove from the oven and let it cool for a few minutes before slicing.

8. Serve the smoked salmon and dill frittata warm or at room temperature.

Buckwheat Banana Pancakes:

- Preparation time: 10 minutes

- Cooking time: 15 minutes

- Servings: 2-3

Ingredients:

- 1 cup buckwheat flour

- 1 tablespoon coconut sugar (or sweetener of choice)

- 1 teaspoon baking powder

- 1/2 teaspoon ground cinnamon

- 1 ripe banana, mashed

- 1 cup almond milk (or any other milk of your choice)

- 1 large egg

- 1 teaspoon vanilla extract

- Coconut oil (for greasing the pan)

- Optional toppings: sliced bananas, maple syrup, chopped nuts

Directions:

1. In a large bowl, whisk together the buckwheat flour, coconut sugar, baking powder, and ground cinnamon.

2. In a separate bowl, combine the mashed banana, almond milk, egg, and vanilla extract. Mix well.

3. Pour the wet ingredients into the dry ingredients and stir until just combined. Do not overmix; a few lumps are okay.

4. Heat a non-stick skillet or griddle over medium heat and lightly grease it with coconut oil.

5. Spoon about 1/4 cup of the pancake batter onto the skillet for each pancake.

6. Cook until the edges are set and bubbles form on the surface, then flip and cook the other side until goldenbrown.

7. Repeat with the remaining batter.

8. Serve the buckwheat banana pancakes warm with your choice of toppings, such as sliced bananas, maple syrup, and chopped nuts.

Tofu Scramble with Vegetables:

- Preparation time: 10 minutes

- Cooking time: 15 minutes

- Servings: 2

Ingredients:

- 1 tablespoon olive oil

- 1/2 onion, diced

- 1 bell pepper, diced

- 2 cloves garlic, minced

- 1/2 teaspoon ground cumin

- 1/2 teaspoon ground turmeric

- 1/4 teaspoon paprika

- Salt and pepper to taste

- 8 ounces firm tofu, drained and crumbled

- 1 cup spinach leaves

- Optional toppings: chopped fresh herbs, sliced avocado, hot sauce

Directions:

1. Heat olive oil in a large skillet over medium heat.

2. Add the diced onion and bell pepper to the skillet and sauté for 5 minutes until softened.

3. Add the minced garlic, ground cumin, ground turmeric, paprika, salt, and pepper. Stir well to coat the vegetables with the spices.

4. Crumble the tofu into the skillet and stir to combine with the vegetables and spices.

5. Cook for about 8 minutes, stirring occasionally, until the tofu is heated through and lightly browned.

6. Add the spinach leaves to the skillet and cook for an additional 2 minutes until wilted.

7. Remove from heat and taste for seasoning, adjusting with salt and pepper if needed.

8. Serve the tofu scramble with vegetables hot, and garnish with optional toppings like chopped fresh herbs, sliced avocado, or hot sauce.

Quiche Lorraine with Gluten-Free Crust:

- Preparation time: 20 minutes

- Cooking time: 40 minutes

- Servings: 6

Ingredients:

For the Crust:

- 1 1/2 cups gluten-free all-purpose flour

- 1/2 teaspoon salt

- 1/2 cup unsalted butter, cold and cubed

- 4-6 tablespoons ice water

For the Filling:

- 6 slices turkey bacon, cooked and crumbled

- 1 cup shredded Gruyere cheese

- 1/2 cup chopped onion

- 4 large eggs

- 1 cup milk

- 1/2 teaspoon salt

- 1/4 teaspoon black pepper

- 1/4 teaspoon ground nutmeg

Directions:

1. Preheat the oven to 375°F (190°C).

2. In a food processor, combine the gluten-free all-purpose flour and salt. Add the cold cubed butter and pulse until the mixture resembles coarse crumbs.

3. Gradually add the ice water, 1 tablespoon at a time, and pulse until the dough comes together.

4. Transfer the dough to a lightly floured surface and roll it out to fit a 9-inch pie dish. Press the dough into the dish and trim any excess.

5. In a bowl, whisk together the eggs, milk, salt, black pepper, and ground nutmeg.

6. Spread the crumbled turkey bacon, shredded Gruyere cheese, and chopped onion evenly over the crust.

7. Pour the egg mixture over the filling ingredients.

8. Bake for about 40 minutes or until the quiche is set and lightly golden.

9. Remove from the oven and let it cool for a few minutes before slicing.

10. Serve the Quiche Lorraine with Gluten-Free Crust warm or at room temperature.

Breakfast Casserole with Turkey Bacon:

- Preparation time: 15 minutes

- Cooking time: 45 minutes

- Servings: 8

Ingredients:

- 8 slices turkey bacon, cooked and crumbled

- 6 large eggs

- 1 1/2 cups milk

- 1 teaspoon Dijon mustard

- 1/2 teaspoon salt

- 1/4 teaspoon black pepper

- 4 cups cubed bread (gluten-free if desired)

- 1 cup shredded cheddar cheese

- 1/2 cup chopped green onions

Directions:

1. Preheat the oven to 375°F (190°C). Grease a 9x13-inch baking dish.

2. In a bowl, whisk together the eggs, milk, Dijon mustard, salt, and black pepper.

3. Place the cubed bread in the prepared baking dish.

4. Sprinkle the crumbled turkey bacon, shredded cheddar cheese, and chopped green onions evenly over the bread.

5. Pour the egg mixture over the ingredients in the baking dish, making sure to coat everything.

6. Press down gently on the ingredients with a spoon to ensure they are submerged in the egg mixture.

7. Cover the baking dish with foil and let it sit in the refrigerator for at least 30 minutes or overnight to allow the bread to absorb the liquid.

8. Remove the foil and bake for about 40-45 minutes or until the casserole is set and golden on top.

9. Remove from the oven and let it cool for a few minutes before serving.

10. Serve the breakfast casserole with turkey bacon warm.

Apple Cinnamon Porridge.

- Preparation time: 5 minutes

- Cooking time: 10 minutes

- Servings: 2

Ingredients:

- 1 cup rolled oats (gluten-free if desired)

- 2 cups almond milk (or any other milk of your choice)

- 1 apple, peeled, cored, and diced

- 1/2 teaspoon ground cinnamon

- 1 tablespoon honey (or sweetener of choice)

- Optional toppings: chopped nuts, raisins, maple syrup

Directions:

1. In a saucepan, combine the rolled oats, almond milk, diced apple, ground cinnamon, and honey.

2. Bring the mixture to a boil over medium heat, then reduce the heat to low.

3. Simmer for about 5-7 minutes, stirring occasionally, until the oats are cooked and the porridge has thickened to your desired consistency.

4. Remove from heat and let it cool for a minute.

5. Serve the apple cinnamon porridge warm, and add optional toppings such as chopped nuts, raisins, or maple syrup.

Cacao and Almond Butter Smoothie:

- Preparation time: 5 minutes

- Servings: 1

Ingredients:

- 1 cup almond milk (or any other milk of your choice)

- 1 ripe banana

- 1 tablespoon almond butter

- 1 tablespoon cacao powder

- 1 tablespoon honey or maple syrup (optional)

- 1/2 teaspoon vanilla extract

- 1/2 cup ice cubes

Directions:

1. In a blender, combine almond milk, ripe banana, almond butter, cacao powder, honey or maple syrup (if desired), vanilla extract, and ice cubes.

2. Blend on high speed until all the ingredients are well combined and the smoothie is creamy and smooth.

3. Taste and adjust the sweetness if needed by adding more honey or maple syrup.

4. Pour the cacao and almond butter smoothie into a glass and serve immediately.

Mediterranean Egg Muffins:

- Preparation time: 10 minutes

- Cooking time: 20 minutes

- Servings: 6

Ingredients:

- 6 large eggs

- 1/4 cup milk

- 1/2 teaspoon dried oregano

- 1/4 teaspoon dried basil

- 1/4 teaspoon dried thyme

- 1/4 teaspoon salt

- 1/4 teaspoon black pepper

- 1/2 cup chopped spinach

- 1/4 cup diced tomatoes

- 1/4 cup chopped bell peppers

- 1/4 cup crumbled feta cheese

Directions:

1. Preheat the oven to 375°F (190°C). Grease a muffin tin or line it with paper liners.

2. In a bowl, whisk together the eggs, milk, dried oregano, dried basil, dried thyme, salt, and black pepper.

3. Divide the chopped spinach, diced tomatoes, chopped bell peppers, and crumbled feta cheese evenly among the muffin cups.

4. Pour the egg mixture over the ingredients in the muffin cups, filling each cup about 3/4 full.

5. Gently stir the ingredients in each cup to ensure they are evenly distributed.

6. Bake for about 18-20 minutes or until the egg muffins are set and lightly golden on top.

7. Remove from the oven and let them cool for a few minutes before removing from the muffin tin.

8. Serve the Mediterranean egg muffins warm or at room temperature.

Chapter 3:

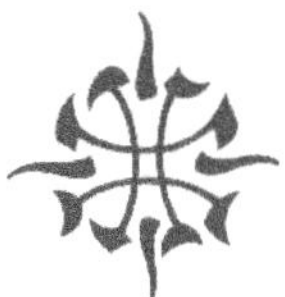

SAVORY SOUPS AND SALADS

Chicken and Vegetable Soup:

- Preparation time: 15 minutes

- Cooking time: 30 minutes

- Servings: 4

Ingredients:

- 1 tablespoon olive oil

- 1 onion, chopped

- 2 carrots, diced

- 2 celery stalks, diced

- 3 cloves garlic, minced

- 4 cups chicken broth

- 2 cups cooked chicken, shredded or diced

- 1 cup diced tomatoes (canned or fresh)

- 1 cup chopped green beans

- 1 teaspoon dried thyme

- 1 bay leaf

- Salt and pepper to taste

- Fresh parsley for garnish (optional)

Directions:

1. Heat the olive oil in a large pot over medium heat.

2. Add the chopped onion, diced carrots, and diced celery. Sauté for about 5 minutes until the vegetables start to soften.

3. Add the minced garlic and sauté for another minute.

4. Pour in the chicken broth and bring to a boil.

5. Reduce the heat to low and add the cooked chicken, diced tomatoes, chopped green beans, dried thyme, and bay leaf.

6. Simmer for about 20 minutes or until the vegetables are tender.

7. Season with salt and pepper to taste.

8. Remove the bay leaf before serving.

9. Garnish with fresh parsley if desired.

10. Serve the chicken and vegetable soup hot.

Nutrition (per serving):

- Calories: 220

- Protein: 20g

- Fat: 7g

- Carbohydrates: 18g

- Fiber: 4g

Quinoa and Kale Salad:

- Preparation time: 15 minutes

- Cooking time: 15 minutes

- Servings: 4

Ingredients:

- 1 cup quinoa

- 2 cups water

- 4 cups kale, stems removed and leaves chopped

- 1 cup cherry tomatoes, halved

- 1/2 cup chopped cucumber

- 1/4 cup chopped red onion

- 1/4 cup chopped fresh parsley

- 1/4 cup crumbled feta cheese

- 2 tablespoons lemon juice

- 2 tablespoons olive oil

- Salt and pepper to taste

Directions:

1. Rinse the quinoa under cold water.

2. In a saucepan, bring the water to a boil. Add the quinoa and reduce the heat to low. Cover and simmer for 12-15 minutes or until the quinoa is cooked and the water is absorbed.

3. In a large bowl, combine the cooked quinoa, chopped kale, cherry tomatoes, chopped cucumber, chopped red onion, and fresh parsley.

4. In a small bowl, whisk together the lemon juice, olive oil, salt, and pepper.

5. Pour the dressing over the salad and toss to combine.

6. Sprinkle the crumbled feta cheese on top.

7. Serve the quinoa and kale salad at room temperature or chilled.

Nutrition (per serving):

- Calories: 240

- Protein: 8g

- Fat: 10g

- Carbohydrates: 32g

- Fiber: 5g

Roasted Butternut Squash Soup:

- Preparation time: 15 minutes

- Cooking time: 45 minutes

- Servings: 6

Ingredients:

- 1 butternut squash, peeled, seeded, and cubed

- 1 onion, chopped

- 2 carrots, chopped

- 2 cloves garlic, minced

- 4 cups vegetable broth

- 1/2 teaspoon ground cinnamon

- 1/4 teaspoon ground nutmeg

- Salt and pepper to taste

- Olive oil for roasting

- Fresh parsley or thyme for garnish (optional)

Directions:

1. Preheat the oven to 400°F (200°C).

2. Place the cubed butternut squash on a baking sheet. Drizzle with olive oil and season with salt and pepper. Toss to coat.

3. Roast the butternut squash in the preheated oven for about 30 minutes or until tender and slightly caramelized.

4. In a large pot, heat some olive oil over medium heat. Add the chopped onion and carrots. Sauté for about 5 minutes until the vegetables start to soften.

5. Add the minced garlic and sauté for another minute.

6. Add the roasted butternut squash, vegetable broth, ground cinnamon, and ground nutmeg to the pot. Bring to a boil.

7. Reduce the heat to low and simmer for about 10 minutes.

8. Use an immersion blender or transfer the soup to a blender and blend until smooth.

9. Season with salt and pepper to taste.

10. Garnish with fresh parsley or thyme if desired.

11. Serve the roasted butternut squash soup hot.

Nutrition (per serving):

- Calories: 130

- Protein: 2g

- Fat: 4g

- Carbohydrates: 25g

- Fiber: 5g

Greek Salad with Grilled Chicken:

- Preparation time: 20 minutes

- Cooking time: 15 minutes (for grilling chicken)

- Servings: 4

Ingredients:

- 2 boneless, skinless chicken breasts

- 1 head romaine lettuce, chopped

- 1 cucumber, seeded and sliced

- 1 cup cherry tomatoes, halved

- 1/2 cup sliced red onion

- 1/2 cup pitted Kalamata olives

- 1/2 cup crumbled feta cheese

- 2 tablespoons extra virgin olive oil

- 2 tablespoons red wine vinegar

- 1 teaspoon dried oregano

- Salt and pepper to taste

Directions:

1. Preheat the grill to medium-high heat.

2. Season the chicken breasts with salt, pepper, and dried oregano.

3. Grill the chicken breasts for about 6-8 minutes per side or until cooked through. Remove from the grill and let them rest for a few minutes. Slice the chicken into strips.

4. In a large salad bowl, combine the chopped romaine lettuce, sliced cucumber, cherry tomatoes, sliced red onion, Kalamata olives, and crumbled feta cheese.

5. In a small bowl, whisk together the extra virgin olive oil, red wine vinegar, dried oregano, salt, and pepper.

6. Drizzle the dressing over the salad and toss to combine.

7. Top the salad with the grilled chicken slices.

8. Serve the Greek salad with grilled chicken immediately.

Nutrition (per serving):

- Calories. 320

- Protein: 28g

- Fat: 18g

- Carbohydrates: 14g

- Fiber: 4g

Tomato and Basil Soup:

- Preparation time: 10 minutes

- Cooking time: 25 minutes

- Servings: 4

Ingredients:

- 2 tablespoons olive oil

- 1 onion, chopped

- 2 cloves garlic, minced

- 4 cups diced tomatoes (canned or fresh)

- 2 cups vegetable broth

- 1/2 cup fresh basil leaves, chopped

- 1/4 cup heavy cream (optional)

- Salt and pepper to taste

- Grated Parmesan cheese for garnish (optional)

Directions:

1. Heat the olive oil in a large pot over medium heat.

2. Add the chopped onion and sauté for about 5 minutes until it becomes translucent.

3. Add the minced garlic and sauté for another minute.

4. Add the diced tomatoes and vegetable broth to the pot. Bring to a boil.

5. Reduce the heat to low and simmer for about 15 minutes.

6. Remove the pot from the heat and let it cool slightly.

7. Use an immersion blender or transfer the soup to a blender and blend until smooth.

8. Return the soup to the pot and stir in the chopped fresh basil leaves.

9. If desired, stir in the heavy cream to make the soup creamy.

10. Season with salt and pepper to taste.

11. Reheat the soup over low heat if necessary.

12. Serve the tomato and basil soup hot.

13. Garnish with grated Parmesan cheese if desired.

Nutrition (per serving):

- Calories: 180

- Protein: 4g

- Fat: 12g

- Carbohydrates: 15g

- Fiber: 4g

Shrimp and Avocado Salad:

- Preparation time: 15 minutes

- Cooking time: 5 minutes

- Servings: 4

Ingredients:

- 1 pound shrimp, peeled and deveined

- 2 avocados, diced

- 1 cup cherry tomatoes, halved

- 1/4 cup red onion, thinly sliced

- 1/4 cup chopped fresh cilantro

- 1 tablespoon olive oil

- 1 tablespoon lime juice

- Salt and pepper to taste

Directions:

1. Heat the olive oil in a skillet over medium heat.

2. Add the shrimp and cook for about 3-4 minutes, until they turn pink and opaque. Remove from heat and let them cool.

3. In a large bowl, combine the diced avocados, cherry tomatoes, red onion, and chopped cilantro.

4. Add the cooked shrimp to the bowl.

5. Drizzle with the olive oil and lime juice.

6. Season with salt and pepper to taste.

7. Gently toss all the ingredients together until well combined.

8. Serve the shrimp and avocado salad immediately.

Nutrition (per serving):

- Calories: 280

- Protein: 25g

- Fat: 15g

- Carbohydrates: 11g

- Fiber: 7g

Carrot and Ginger Soup:

- Preparation time: 15 minutes

- Cooking time: 25 minutes

- Servings: 4

Ingredients:

- 1 tablespoon olive oil

- 1 onion, chopped

- 3 cloves garlic, minced

- 1 pound carrots, peeled and chopped

- 1 tablespoon grated fresh ginger

- 4 cups vegetable broth

- 1/2 cup coconut milk

- Salt and pepper to taste

- Chopped fresh cilantro or parsley for garnish (optional)

Directions:

1. Heat the olive oil in a large pot over medium heat.

2. Add the chopped onion and sauté for about 5 minutes until it becomes translucent.

3. Add the minced garlic and grated ginger. Sauté for another minute.

4. Add the chopped carrots and vegetable broth to the pot. Bring to a boil.

5. Reduce the heat to low and simmer for about 20 minutes or until the carrots are tender.

6. Remove the pot from the heat and let it cool slightly.

7. Use an immersion blender or transfer the soup to a blender and blend until smooth.

8. Return the soup to the pot. Stir in the coconut milk.

9. Season with salt and pepper to taste.

10. Reheat the soup over low heat if necessary.

11. Serve the carrot and ginger soup hot.

12. Garnish with chopped fresh cilantro or parsley if desired.

Nutrition (per serving):

- Calories: 150

- Protein: 2g

- Fat: 9g

- Carbohydrates: 16g

- Fiber: 4g

Spinach and Strawberry Salad:

- Preparation time: 10 minutes

- Servings: 4

Ingredients:

- 6 cups baby spinach leaves

- 1 cup sliced strawberries

- 1/4 cup sliced almonds

- 1/4 cup crumbled feta cheese

- 2 tablespoons balsamic vinegar

- 2 tablespoons extra virgin olive oil

- 1 tablespoon honey

- Salt and pepper to taste

Directions:

1. In a large salad bowl, combine the baby spinach leaves, sliced strawberries, sliced almonds, and crumbled feta cheese.

2. In a small bowl, whisk together the balsamic vinegar, extra virgin olive oil, honey, salt, and pepper.

3. Drizzle the dressing over the salad.

4. Toss gently to coat the ingredients with the dressing.

5. Serve the spinach and strawberry salad immediately.

Nutrition (per serving):

- Calories: 150

- Protein: 4g

- Fat: 10g

- Carbohydrates: 13g

- Fiber: 4g

Cauliflower and Leek Soup:

- Preparation time: 15 minutes

- Cooking time: 25 minutes

- Servings: 4

Ingredients:

- 1 tablespoon olive oil

- 2 leeks, white and light green parts only, sliced

- 1 head cauliflower, chopped into florets

- 2 cloves garlic, minced

- 4 cups vegetable broth

- 1/2 cup heavy cream (optional)

- Salt and pepper to taste

- Chopped fresh chives or parsley for garnish (optional)

Directions:

1. Heat the olive oil in a large pot over medium heat.

2. Add the sliced leeks and sauté for about 5 minutes until they become soft.

3. Add the chopped cauliflower florets and minced garlic. Sauté for another minute.

4. Pour in the vegetable broth and bring to a boil.

5. Reduce the heat to low andsimmer for about 20 minutes or until the cauliflower is tender.

6. Remove the pot from the heat and let it cool slightly.

7. Use an immersion blender or transfer the soup to a blender and blend until smooth.

8. Return the soup to the pot. Stir in the heavy cream, if using.

9. Season with salt and pepper to taste.

10. Reheat the soup over low heat if necessary.

11. Serve the cauliflower and leek soup hot.

12. Garnish with chopped fresh chives or parsley if desired.

Nutrition (per serving):

- Calories: 180

- Protein: 5g

- Fat: 13g

- Carbohydrates: 14g

- Fiber: 5g

Caprese Salad with Balsamic Glaze:

- Preparation time: 10 minutes

- Servings: 4

Ingredients:

- 3 large tomatoes, sliced

- 8 ounces fresh mozzarella cheese, sliced

- 1/2 cup fresh basil leaves

- 2 tablespoons balsamic glaze

- 2 tablespoons extra virgin olive oil

- Salt and pepper to taste

Directions:

1. Arrange the tomato slices on a serving platter.

2. Place a slice of mozzarella on each tomato slice.

3. Top each mozzarella slice with a fresh basil leaf.

4. Drizzle the balsamic glaze and extra virgin olive oil over the salad.

5. Season with salt and pepper to taste.

6. Serve the Caprese salad immediately.

Nutrition (per serving):

- Calories: 220

- Protein: 11g

- Fat: 17g

- Carbohydrates: 7g

- Fiber: 1g

Zucchini and Corn Chowder:

- Preparation time: 15 minutes

- Cooking time: 25 minutes

- Servings: 4

Ingredients:

- 2 tablespoons butter or olive oil

- 1 onion, chopped

- 2 cloves garlic, minced

- 2 zucchinis, diced

- 2 cups corn kernels (fresh or frozen)

- 4 cups vegetable broth

- 1 cup milk or cream

- 1 teaspoon dried thyme

- Salt and pepper to taste

- Chopped fresh parsley for garnish (optional)

Directions:

1. Heat the butter or olive oil in a large pot over medium heat.

2. Add the chopped onion and sauté for about 5 minutes until it becomes translucent.

3. Add the minced garlic and diced zucchinis. Sauté for another 2-3 minutes.

4. Add the corn kernels, vegetable broth, and dried thyme to the pot. Bring to a boil.

5. Reduce the heat to low and simmer for about 15 minutes or until the zucchini is tender.

6. Use an immersion blender or transfer about half of the soup to a blender and blend until smooth.

7. Return the blended soup to the pot.

8. Stir in the milk or cream. Season with salt and pepper to taste.

9. Reheat the soup over low heat if necessary.

10. Serve the zucchini and corn chowder hot.

11. Garnish with chopped fresh parsley if desired.

Nutrition (per serving):

- Calories: 220

- Protein: 7g

- Fat: 10g

- Carbohydrates: 30g

- Fiber: 5g

Quinoa and Black Bean Salad:

- Preparation time: 15 minutes

- Cooking time: 15 minutes

- Servings: 4

Ingredients:

- 1 cup quinoa

- 2 cups water

- 1 can (15 ounces) black beans, rinsed and drained

- 1 red bell pepper, diced

- 1 cup cherry tomatoes, halved

- 1/4 cup chopped red onion

- 1/4 cup chopped fresh cilantro

- Juice of 1 lime

- 2 tablespoons extra virgin olive oil

- Salt and pepper to taste

- Optional: avocado slices for garnish

Directions:

1. Rinse the quinoa under cold water.

2. In a saucepan, bring the water to a boil. Add the rinsed quinoa and reduce the heat to low.

3. Cover the saucepan and simmer for about 15 minutes or until the quinoa is cooked and the water is absorbed.

4. Remove the saucepan from the heat and let the quinoa cool.

5. In a large bowl, combine the cooked quinoa, black beans, diced red bell pepper, cherry tomatoes, chopped red onion, and chopped cilantro.

6. In a small bowl, whisk together the lime juice, extra virgin olive oil, salt, and pepper.

7. Drizzle the dressing over the salad.

8. Toss gently to coat all the ingredients with the dressing.

9. Serve the quinoa and black bean salad at room temperature or chilled.

10. Garnish with avocado slices if desired.

Nutrition (per serving):

- Calories: 320

- Protein: 12g

- Fat: 10g

- Carbohydrates: 48g

- Fiber: 12g

Creamy Broccoli Soup:

- Preparation time: 10 minutes

- Cooking time: 20 minutes

- Servings: 4

Ingredients:

- 2 tablespoons butter or olive oil

- 1 onion, chopped

- 2 cloves garlic, minced

- 4 cups chopped broccoli florets

- 4 cups vegetable broth

- 1 cup milk or cream

- Salt and pepper to taste

- Grated cheddar cheese for garnish (optional)

Directions:

1. Heat the butter or olive oil in a large pot over medium heat.

2. Add the chopped onion and sauté for about 5 minutes until it becomes translucent.

3. Add the minced garlic and chopped broccoli florets. Sauté for another 2-3 minutes.

4. Pour in the vegetable broth and bring to a boil.

5. Reduce the heat to low and simmer for about 15 minutes or until the broccoli is tender.

6. Use an immersion blender or transfer about half of the soup to a blender and blend until smooth.

7. Return the blended soup to the pot.

8. Stir in the milk or cream. Season with salt and pepper to taste.

9. Reheat the soup over low heat if necessary.

10. Serve the creamy broccoli soup hot.

11. Garnish with grated cheddar cheese if desired.

Nutrition (per serving):

- Calories: 180

- Protein: 6g

- Fat: 10g

- Carbohydrates: 20g

- Fiber: 5g

Watermelon and Feta Salad:

- Preparation time: 10 minutes

- Servings: 4

Ingredients:

- 4 cups cubed watermelon

- 1 cup crumbled feta cheese

- 1/4 cup fresh mint leaves, torn

- 2 tablespoons extra virgin olive oil

- 1 tablespoon balsamic vinegar

- Salt and pepper to taste

Directions:

1. In a large bowl, combine the cubed watermelon, crumbled feta cheese, and torn mint leaves.

2. In a small bowl, whisk together the extra virgin olive oil, balsamic vinegar, salt, and pepper.

3. Drizzle the dressing over the watermelon and feta salad.

4. Toss gently to coat the ingredients with the dressing.

5. Serve the salad immediately or refrigerate for later use.

Nutrition (per serving):

- Calories: 180

- Protein: 6g

- Fat: 12g

- Carbohydrates: 14g

- Fiber: 1g

Lentil Soup with Vegetables:

- Preparation time: 15 minutes

- Cooking time: 40 minutes

- Servings: 6

Ingredients:

- 1 cup dried lentils, rinsed and drained

- 6 cups vegetable broth

- 1 onion, chopped

- 2 carrots, diced

- 2 celery stalks, diced

- 2 cloves garlic, minced

- 1 teaspoon ground cumin

- 1 teaspoon ground coriander

- 1 bay leaf

- 2 tablespoons olive oil

- Salt and pepper to taste

- Chopped fresh parsley for garnish (optional)

Directions:

1. In a large pot, heat the olive oil over medium heat.

2. Add the chopped onion, diced carrots, diced celery, and minced garlic. Sauté for about 5 minutes until the vegetables soften.

3. Add the ground cumin, ground coriander, and bay leaf. Stir to coat the vegetables with the spices.

4. Add the rinsed lentils and vegetable broth to the pot. Bring to a boil.

5. Reduce the heat to low and simmer for about 30-35 minutes or until the lentils are tender.

6. Remove the bay leaf from the soup.

7. Season with salt and pepper to taste.

8. Serve the lentil soup with vegetables hot.

9. Garnish with chopped fresh parsley if desired.

Nutrition (per serving):

- Calories: 220

- Protein: 12g

- Fat: 5g

- Carbohydrates: 32g

- Fiber: 10g

Asian Cucumber Salad:

- Preparation time: 10 minutes

- Servings: 4

Ingredients:

- 2 cucumbers, thinly sliced

- 1 carrot, julienned

- 1/4 cup rice vinegar

- 1 tablespoon soy sauce

- 1 tablespoon sesame oil

- 1 tablespoon honey or maple syrup

- 1 teaspoon grated ginger

- 2 tablespoons chopped fresh cilantro

- Sesame seeds for garnish (optional)

Directions:

1. In a large bowl, combine the sliced cucumbers and julienned carrot.

2. In a separate small bowl, whisk together the rice vinegar, soy sauce, sesame oil, honey or maple syrup, and grated ginger.

3. Pour the dressing over the cucumber and carrot mixture.

4. Toss gently to coat the vegetables with the dressing.

5. Sprinkle with chopped fresh cilantro and sesame seeds.

6. Serve the Asian cucumber salad chilled.

Nutrition (per serving):

- Calories: 60

- Protein: 1g

- Fat: 3g

- Carbohydrates: 9g

- Fiber: 2g

Creamy Mushroom Soup:

- Preparation time: 10 minutes

- Cooking time: 25 minutes

- Servings: 4

Ingredients:

- 1 pound mushrooms, sliced

- 1 onion, chopped

- 2 cloves garlic, minced

- 2 tablespoons butter or olive oil

- 4 cups vegetable broth

- 1 cup heavy cream or coconut cream

- 1 teaspoon dried thyme

- Salt and pepper to taste

- Chopped fresh parsley for garnish (optional)

Directions:

1. In a large pot, melt the butter or heat the olive oil over medium heat.

2. Add the chopped onion and sauté for about 5 minutes until it becomes translucent.

3. Add the minced garlic and sliced mushrooms. Sauté for another 5-7 minutes until the mushrooms are cooked.

4. Pour in the vegetable broth and add the dried thyme. Bring to a boil.

5. Reduce the heat to low and simmer for about 10 minutes.

6. Use an immersion blender or transfer about half of the soup to a blender and blend until smooth.

7. Return the blended soup to the pot.

8. Stir in the heavy cream or coconut cream. Season with salt and pepper to taste.

9. Reheat the soup over low heat if necessary.

10. Serve the creamy mushroom soup hot.

11. Garnish with chopped fresh parsley if desired.

Nutrition (per serving):

- Calories: 220

- Protein: 4g

- Fat: 18g

- Carbohydrates: 11g

- Fiber: 2g

Quinoa Tabouli Salad:

- Preparation time: 15 minutes

- Cooking time: 15 minutes

- Servings: 4

Ingredients:

- 1 cup cooked quinoa

- 1 cucumber, diced

- 2 tomatoes, diced

- 1/2 cup finely chopped fresh parsley

- 1/4 cup chopped fresh mint leaves

- 1/4 cup chopped red onion

- Juice of 1 lemon

- 2 tablespoons extra virgin olive oil

- Salt and pepper to taste

Directions:

1. In a large bowl, combine the cooked quinoa, diced cucumber, diced tomatoes, chopped fresh parsley, chopped fresh mint leaves, and chopped red onion.

2. In a small bowl, whisk together the lemon juice, extra virgin olive oil, salt, and pepper.

3. Drizzle the dressing over the quinoa tabouli salad.

4. Toss gently to coat all the ingredients with the dressing.

5. Serve the salad at room temperature or chilled.

Nutrition (per serving):

- Calories: 180

- Protein: 6g

- Fat: 8g

- Carbohydrates: 24g

- Fiber: 4g

Roasted Red Pepper Soup:

- Preparation time: 10 minutes

- Cooking time: 40 minutes

- Servings: 4

Ingredients:

- 3 red bell peppers

- 1 onion, chopped

- 2 cloves garlic, minced

- 2 tablespoons olive oil

- 4 cups vegetable broth

- 1 can (14 ounces) diced tomatoes

- 1 teaspoon smoked paprika

- Salt and pepper to taste

- Chopped fresh basil for garnish (optional)

Directions:

1. Preheat the oven to 425°F (220°C).

2. Cut the red bell peppers in half and remove the seeds and stems.

3. Place the pepper halves on a baking sheet, cut side down.

4. Roast the peppers in the preheated oven for about 20-25 minutes or until the skins are charred and blistered.

5. Remove the peppers from the oven and let them cool. Once cooled, peelthe skins off the peppers and chop them into smaller pieces.

6. In a large pot, heat the olive oil over medium heat.

7. Add the chopped onion and minced garlic, and sauté for about 5 minutes until the onion becomes translucent.

8. Add the roasted red peppers, vegetable broth, diced tomatoes (with their juices), smoked paprika, salt, and pepper to the pot.

9. Bring the mixture to a boil, then reduce the heat to low and simmer for about 15 minutes.

10. Use an immersion blender or transfer the soup to a blender and blend until smooth.

11. Return the blended soup to the pot and reheat over low heat if necessary.

12. Serve the roasted red pepper soup hot.

13. Garnish with chopped fresh basil if desired.

Nutrition (per serving):

- Calories: 140

- Protein: 3g

- Fat: 8g

- Carbohydrates: 15g

- Fiber: 4g

Greek Orzo Salad:

- Preparation time: 15 minutes

- Cooking time: 10 minutes

- Servings: 4

Ingredients:

- 1 cup orzo pasta

- 1 English cucumber, diced

- 1 cup cherry tomatoes, halved

- 1/2 red onion, thinly sliced

- 1/2 cup Kalamata olives, pitted and halved

- 1/2 cup crumbled feta cheese

- 1/4 cup chopped fresh parsley

- 2 tablespoons extra virgin olive oil

- Juice of 1 lemon

- Salt and pepper to taste

Directions:

1. Cook the orzo pasta according to the package instructions. Drain and rinse with cold water.

2. In a large bowl, combine the cooked orzo pasta, diced cucumber, halved cherry tomatoes, thinly sliced red onion, halved Kalamata olives, crumbled feta cheese, and chopped fresh parsley.

3. In a small bowl, whisk together the extra virgin olive oil, lemon juice, salt, and pepper.

4. Drizzle the dressing over the Greek orzo salad.

5. Toss gently to coat all the ingredients with the dressing.

6. Serve the salad at room temperature or chilled.

Nutrition (per serving):

- Calories: 280

- Protein: 8g

- Fat: 12g

- Carbohydrates: 35g

- Fiber: 3g

Chapter 4:

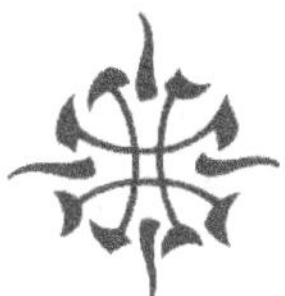

DELECTABLE ENTREES

Baked Salmon with Lemon and Dill:

- Preparation time: 10 minutes

- Cooking time: 15-20 minutes

- Servings: 4

Ingredients:

- 4 salmon fillets

- 2 tablespoons fresh lemon juice

- 2 tablespoons olive oil

- 2 cloves garlic, minced

- 1 tablespoon chopped fresh dill

- Salt and pepper to taste

- Lemon slices for garnish (optional)

Directions:

1. Preheat the oven to 400°F (200°C) and line a baking sheet with parchment paper.

2. In a small bowl, whisk together the lemon juice, olive oil, minced garlic, chopped fresh dill, salt, and pepper.

3. Place the salmon fillets on the prepared baking sheet.

4. Drizzle the lemon and dill mixture over the salmon, making sure it is evenly coated.

5. Bake the salmon in the preheated oven for 15-20 minutes, or until it flakes easily with a fork.

6. Serve the baked salmon with lemon and dill hot.

7. Garnish with lemon slices if desired.

Nutrition (per serving):

- Calories: 300

- Protein: 34g

- Fat: 17g

- Carbohydrates: 1g

- Fiber: 0g

Grilled Chicken with Rosemary and Garlic:

- Preparation time: 10 minutes

- Cooking time: 15-20 minutes

- Servings: 4

Ingredients:

- 4 boneless, skinless chicken breasts

- 2 tablespoons olive oil

- 2 cloves garlic, minced

- 1 tablespoon chopped fresh rosemary

- Salt and pepper to taste

- Lemon wedges for serving (optional)

Directions:

1. Preheat the grill to medium-high heat.

2. In a small bowl, combine the olive oil, minced garlic, chopped fresh rosemary, salt, and pepper.

3. Brush the chicken breasts with the rosemary and garlic mixture, coating both sides.

4. Place the chicken breasts on the preheated grill and cook for 6-8 minutes per side, or until the internal temperature reaches 165°F (74°C).

5. Remove the chicken from the grill and let it rest for a few minutes before serving.

6. Serve the grilled chicken with rosemary and garlic hot.

7. Squeeze lemon wedges over the chicken if desired.

Nutrition (per serving):

- Calories: 220

- Protein: 32g

- Fat: 9g

- Carbohydrates: 1g

- Fiber: 0g

Quinoa-Stuffed Bell Peppers:

- Preparation time: 15 minutes

- Cooking time: 40 minutes

- Servings: 4

Ingredients:

- 4 bell peppers (any color)

- 1 cup cooked quinoa

- 1 cup canned black beans, rinsed and drained

- 1 cup corn kernels (fresh or frozen)

- 1/2 cup diced tomatoes

- 1/2 cup shredded cheddar cheese (optional)

- 2 tablespoons chopped fresh cilantro

- 1 teaspoon ground cumin

- 1/2 teaspoon chili powder

- Salt and pepper to taste

Directions:

1. Preheat the oven to 375°F (190°C) and lightly grease a baking dish.

2. Cut the tops off the bell peppers and remove the seeds and membranes.

3. In a large bowl, combine the cooked quinoa, black beans, corn kernels, diced tomatoes, shredded cheddar cheese (if using), chopped fresh cilantro, ground cumin, chili powder, salt, and pepper. Mix well.

4. Spoon the quinoa mixture into the hollowed-out bell peppers, packing it tightly.

5. Place the stuffed bell peppers in the prepared baking dish.

6. Cover the dish with foil and bake in the preheated oven for 25 minutes.

7. Remove the foil and bake for an additional 10-15 minutes, or until the bell peppers are tender and the filling is heated through.

8. Serve the quinoa-stuffed bell peppers hot.

Nutrition (per serving):

- Calories: 240

- Protein: 11g

- Fat: 4g

- Carbohydrates: 44g

- Fiber: 10g

Shrimp Stir-Fry with Veggies:

- Preparation time: 10 minutes

- Cooking time: 10 minutes

- Servings: 4

Ingredients:

- 1 pound shrimp, peeled and deveined

- 2 tablespoons soy sauce

- 2 tablespoons oyster sauce

- 1 tablespoon sesame oil

- 1 tablespoon cornstarch

- 1 tablespoon vegetable oil

- 2 cloves garlic, minced

- 1-inch piece of ginger, grated

- 1 bell pepper, thinly sliced

- 1 carrot, julienned

- 1 cup broccoli florets

- 1 cup snap peas

- Salt and pepper to taste

- Cooked rice for serving

Directions:

1. In a small bowl, whisk together the soy sauce, oyster sauce, sesame oil, and cornstarch. Set aside.

2. Heat the vegetable oil in a large skillet or wok over medium-high heat.

3. Add the minced garlic and grated ginger to the skillet and sauté for 1 minute until fragrant.

4. Add the shrimp to the skillet and cook for 2-3 minutes until they start to turn pink.

5. Add the sliced bell pepper, julienned carrot, broccoli florets, and snap peas to the skillet. Stir-fry for 3-4 minutes until the vegetables are crisp-tender.

6. Pour the sauce mixture over the shrimp and vegetables in the skillet. Stir well to coat everything evenly.

7. Cook for another 2-3 minutes until the sauce thickens and coats the shrimp and vegetables.

8. Season with salt and pepper to taste.

9. Serve the shrimp stir-fry with veggies over cooked rice.

Nutrition (per serving):

- Calories: 250

- Protein: 25g

- Fat: 10g

- Carbohydrates: 15g

- Fiber: 3g

Baked Cod with Herbs and Lemon:

- Preparation time: 10 minutes

- Cooking time: 15 minutes

- Servings: 4

Ingredients:

- 4 cod fillets

- 2 tablespoons olive oil

- 2 cloves garlic, minced

- 1 tablespoon chopped fresh parsley

- 1 teaspoon chopped fresh thyme

- 1 teaspoon chopped fresh rosemary

- 1 lemon, sliced

- Salt and pepper to taste

Directions:

1. Preheat the oven to 400°F (200°C) and line a baking sheet with parchment paper.

2. Place the cod fillets on the prepared baking sheet.

3. In a small bowl, combine the olive oil, minced garlic, chopped fresh parsley, chopped fresh thyme, chopped fresh rosemary, salt, and pepper.

4. Drizzle the herb and garlic mixture over the cod fillets, making sure they are evenly coated.

5. Place lemon slices on top of each cod fillet.

6. Bake in the preheated oven for 15 minutes, or until the cod is cooked through and flakes easily with a fork.

7. Serve the baked cod with herbs and lemon hot.

Nutrition (per serving):

- Calories: 180

- Protein: 30g

- Fat: 6g

- Carbohydrates: 2g

- Fiber: 0g

Turkey Meatballs with Zucchini Noodles:

- Preparation time: 15 minutes

- Cooking time: 25 minutes

- Servings: 4

Ingredients:

- 1 pound ground turkey

- 1/4 cup breadcrumbs

- 1/4 cup grated Parmesan cheese

- 1/4 cup chopped fresh parsley

- 1 egg

- 2 cloves garlic, minced

- 1/2 teaspoon dried oregano

- Salt and pepper to taste

- 2 tablespoons olive oil

- 4 medium zucchini, spiralized into noodles

- 2 cups marinara sauce

Directions:

1. In a large bowl, combine the ground turkey, breadcrumbs, grated Parmesan cheese, chopped fresh parsley, egg, minced garlic, dried oregano, salt, and pepper. Mix well.

2. Shape the turkey mixture into meatballs, about 1 inch in diameter.

3. Heat the olive oil in a large skillet over medium heat. Add the turkey meatballs and cook for 8-10 minutes, or until browned on all sides and cooked through.

4. Remove the turkey meatballs from the skillet and set aside.

5. In the same skillet, add the spiralized zucchini noodles and cook for 2-3 minutes until tender.

6. Pour the marinara sauce into the skillet with the zucchini noodles and stir to combine.

7. Return the turkey meatballs to the skillet and simmer for another 5 minutes to heat through.

8. Serve the turkey meatballs with zucchini noodles hot.

Nutrition (per serving):

- Calories: 350

- Protein: 27g

- Fat: 18g

- Carbohydrates: 22g

- Fiber: 5g

Eggplant Parmesan with Gluten-Free Breadcrumbs:

- Preparation time: 20 minutes

- Cooking time: 40 minutes

- Servings: 4

Ingredients:

- 2 large eggplants, cut into 1/4-inch thick slices

- Salt

- 1 cup gluten-free breadcrumbs

- 1/2 cup grated Parmesan cheese

- 2 teaspoons dried Italian seasoning

- 2 eggs, beaten

- Olive oil for frying

- 2 cups marinara sauce

- 1 cup shredded mozzarella cheese

- Fresh basil leaves for garnish (optional)

Directions:

1. Sprinkle the eggplant slices with salt and let them sit for 15 minutes to remove excess moisture. Pat dry with paper towels.

2. In a shallow dish, combine the gluten-free breadcrumbs, grated Parmesan cheese, and dried Italian seasoning.

3. Dip each eggplant slice into the beaten eggs, then coat it with the breadcrumb mixture, pressing gently to adhere.

4. Heat olive oil in a large skillet over medium heat. Fry the breaded eggplant slices in batches for about 2-3 minutes per side, or until golden brown. Drain on paper towels.

5. Preheat the oven to 375°F (190°C). Spread a thin layer of marinara sauce on the bottom of a baking dish.

6. Arrange a single layer of fried eggplant slices in the baking dish, slightly overlapping. Top with more marinara sauce and shredded mozzarella cheese.

7. Repeat the layers until all the eggplant slices are used, finishing with marinara sauce and mozzarella cheese on top.

8. Bake in the preheated oven for 20-25 minutes, or until the cheese is melted and bubbly.

9. Let the eggplant Parmesan cool for a few minutes before serving.

10. Garnish with fresh basil leaves if desired.

Nutrition (per serving):

- Calories: 380

- Protein: 16g

- Fat: 18g

- Carbohydrates: 43g

- Fiber: 12g

Lemon Herb Roasted Chicken Thighs:

- Preparation time: 10 minutes

- Cooking time: 30 minutes

- Servings: 4

Ingredients:

- 4 chicken thighs, bone-in and skin-on

- 2 tablespoons olive oil

- 2 tablespoons fresh lemon juice

- 2 cloves garlic, minced

- 1 tablespoon chopped fresh thyme

- 1 tablespoon chopped fresh rosemary

- Salt and pepper to taste

- Lemon slices for garnish (optional)

Directions:

1. Preheat the oven to 425°F (220°C) and line a baking sheet with parchment paper.

2. In a small bowl, whisk together the olive oil, lemon juice, minced garlic, chopped fresh thyme, chopped fresh rosemary, salt, and pepper.

3. Place the chicken thighs on the prepared baking sheet.

4. Drizzle the lemon herb mixture over the chicken thighs, making sure they are evenly coated.

5. Place lemon slices on top of each chicken thigh.

6. Roast in the preheated oven for 25-30 minutes, or until the chicken is cooked through andthe skin is crispy and golden brown.

7. Remove from the oven and let the chicken thighs rest for a few minutes before serving.

8. Serve the lemon herb roasted chicken thighs with your choice of sides.

Nutrition (per serving):

- Calories: 350

- Protein: 21g

- Fat: 27g

- Carbohydrates: 2g

- Fiber: 0g

Stuffed Portobello Mushrooms with Quinoa and Spinach:

- Preparation time: 15 minutes

- Cooking time: 25 minutes

- Servings: 4

Ingredients:

- 4 large Portobello mushrooms

- 1 cup cooked quinoa

- 1 cup chopped spinach

- 1/2 cup diced onion

- 2 cloves garlic, minced

- 1/2 cup shredded mozzarella cheese

- 2 tablespoons grated Parmesan cheese

- 2 tablespoons olive oil

- Salt and pepper to taste

Directions:

1. Preheat the oven to 375°F (190°C) and line a baking sheet with parchment paper.

2. Remove the stems from the Portobello mushrooms and gently scrape out the gills with a spoon.

3. In a large skillet, heat the olive oil over medium heat. Add the diced onion and minced garlic, and sauté until the onion is translucent and fragrant.

4. Add the chopped spinach to the skillet and cook until wilted.

5. In a bowl, combine the cooked quinoa, sautéed onion, garlic, and spinach. Season with salt and pepper to taste.

6. Spoon the quinoa mixture into the Portobello mushroom caps, dividing it evenly.

7. Sprinkle the shredded mozzarella cheese and grated Parmesan cheese on top of each stuffed mushroom.

8. Place the stuffed Portobello mushrooms on the prepared baking sheet and bake in the preheated oven for 20-25 minutes, or until the mushrooms are tender and the cheese is melted and golden brown.

9. Remove from the oven and let the stuffed mushrooms cool for a few minutes before serving.

Nutrition (per serving):

- Calories: 220

- Protein: 11g

- Fat: 11g

- Carbohydrates: 21g

- Fiber: 4g

Baked Tofu with Asian Glaze:

- Preparation time: 10 minutes

- Cooking time: 25 minutes

- Servings: 4

Ingredients:

- 1 block firm tofu, drained and pressed

- 2 tablespoons soy sauce

- 2 tablespoons hoisin sauce

- 1 tablespoon rice vinegar

- 1 tablespoon honey or maple syrup

- 1 clove garlic, minced

- 1 teaspoon grated fresh ginger

- 1 tablespoon sesame oil

- 1 tablespoon sesame seeds (optional)

- Chopped green onions for garnish (optional)

Directions:

1. Preheat the oven to 400°F (200°C) and line a baking sheet with parchment paper.

2. Cut the pressed tofu into cubes or slices, depending on your preference.

3. In a small bowl, whisk together the soy sauce, hoisin sauce, rice vinegar, honey or maple syrup, minced garlic, grated fresh ginger, and sesame oil.

4. Place the tofu on the prepared baking sheet and drizzle the Asian glaze over the tofu, making sure each piece is coated.

5. Sprinkle sesame seeds on top of the tofu if desired.

6. Bake in the preheated oven for 25 minutes, or until the tofu is golden brown and slightly crispy.

7. Remove from the oven and let the baked tofu cool for a few minutes before serving.

8. Garnish with chopped green onions if desired.

Nutrition (per serving):

- Calories: 180

- Protein: 12g

- Fat: 10g

- Carbohydrates: 14g

- Fiber: 2g

Beef Stir-Fry with Broccoli and Snow Peas:

- Preparation time: 15 minutes

- Cooking time: 15 minutes

- Servings: 4

Ingredients:

- 1 pound beef steak (such as sirloin or flank), thinly sliced

- 2 tablespoons soy sauce

- 1 tablespoon oyster sauce

- 1 tablespoon cornstarch

- 2 tablespoons vegetable oil

- 2 cloves garlic, minced

- 1 teaspoon grated fresh ginger

- 2 cups broccoli florets

- 1 cup snow peas

- 1/2 cup sliced carrots

- Salt and pepper to taste

- Cooked rice or noodles for serving

Directions:

1. In a bowl, combine the sliced beef, soy sauce, oyster sauce, and cornstarch. Mix until the beef is well-coated. Set aside.

2. Heat the vegetable oil in a large skillet or wok over high heat.

3. Add the minced garlic and grated ginger to the skillet and stir-fry for about 30 seconds, until fragrant.

4. Add the marinated beef to the skillet and stir-fry for 2-3 minutes, until browned.

5. Add the broccoli florets, snow peas, and sliced carrots to the skillet. Stir-fry for another 3-4 minutes, until the vegetables are crisp-tender.

6. Season with salt and pepper to taste.

7. Serve the beef stir-fry with broccoli and snow peas over cooked rice or noodles.

Nutrition (per serving):

- Calories: 320

- Protein: 25g

- Fat: 16g

- Carbohydrates: 20g

- Fiber: 5g

Cauliflower "Steak" with Chimichurri Sauce:

- Preparation time: 10 minutes

- Cooking time: 25 minutes

- Servings: 4

Ingredients:

- 1 large head cauliflower

- 3 tablespoons olive oil

- Salt and pepper to taste

- 1/2 cup chopped fresh parsley

- 3 tablespoons chopped fresh cilantro

- 2 tablespoons chopped fresh oregano

- 2 cloves garlic, minced

- 2 tablespoons red wine vinegar

- 1/4 cup olive oil

- Juice of 1/2 lemon

- Salt and pepper to taste

Directions:

1. Preheat the oven to 425°F (220°C) and line a baking sheet with parchment paper.

2. Remove the leaves from the cauliflower and trim the stem end, leaving the core intact.

3. Slice the cauliflower into 1-inch thick "steaks."

4. Place the cauliflower steaks on the prepared baking sheet and brush both sides with olive oil. Season with salt and pepper to taste.

5. Roast in the preheated oven for 20-25 minutes, flipping the steaks halfway through, until the cauliflower is tender and golden brown.

6. While the cauliflower is roasting, prepare the chimichurri sauce. In a bowl, combine the chopped parsley, chopped cilantro, chopped oregano, minced garlic, red wine vinegar, olive oil, lemon juice, salt, and pepper. Mix well.

7. Remove the roasted cauliflower steaks from the oven and let them cool for a few minutes.

8. Serve the cauliflower "steaks" with the chimichurri sauce drizzled on top.

Nutrition (per serving):

- Calories: 180

- Protein: 5g

- Fat: 16g

- Carbohydrates: 9g

- Fiber: 4g

Lentil Curry with Coconut Milk:

- Preparation time: 15 minutes

- Cooking time: 30 minutes

- Servings: 4

Ingredients:

- 1 cup dried lentils (any variety), rinsed

- 1 tablespoon vegetable oil

- 1 onion, chopped

- 2 cloves garlic, minced

- 1 tablespoon grated fresh ginger

- 2 tablespoons curry powder

- 1 teaspoon ground cumin

- 1/2 teaspoon ground turmeric

- 1 can (14 ounces) coconut milk

- 1 can (14 ounces) diced tomatoes

- 2 cups vegetable broth

- 2 cups chopped vegetables (such as carrots, bell peppers, or cauliflower)

- Salt and pepper to taste

- Cooked rice or naan bread for serving

Directions:

1. In a large pot, heat the vegetable oil over medium heat.

2. Add the chopped onion to the pot and sauté for 3-4 minutes, until softened.

3. Add the minced garlic and grated ginger to the pot and sauté for another 1 minute, until fragrant.

4. Stir in the curry powder, ground cumin, and ground turmeric, and cook for 1 minute to toast the spices.

5. Add the rinsed lentils, coconut milk, diced tomatoes (with theirjuices), vegetable broth, and chopped vegetables to the pot. Stir to combine.

6. Bring the mixture to a boil, then reduce the heat to low, cover the pot, and simmer for 25-30 minutes, or until the lentils and vegetables are tender.

7. Season with salt and pepper to taste.

8. Serve the lentil curry over cooked rice or with naan bread.

Nutrition (per serving):

- Calories: 320

- Protein: 13g

- Fat: 12g

- Carbohydrates: 42g

- Fiber: 15g

Turkey Chili with Black Beans:

- Preparation time: 15 minutes

- Cooking time: 45 minutes

- Servings: 6

Ingredients:

- 1 tablespoon olive oil

- 1 pound ground turkey

- 1 onion, chopped

- 2 cloves garlic, minced

- 1 bell pepper, chopped

- 1 can (14 ounces) diced tomatoes

- 1 can (14 ounces) tomato sauce

- 1 can (14 ounces) black beans, rinsed and drained

- 1 cup corn kernels

- 2 tablespoons chili powder

- 1 teaspoon ground cumin

- 1/2 teaspoon paprika

- 1/2 teaspoon dried oregano

- Salt and pepper to taste

- Optional toppings: shredded cheese, sour cream, chopped green onions

Directions:

1. In a large pot, heat the olive oil over medium heat.

2. Add the ground turkey to the pot and cook, breaking it up with a spoon, until browned and cooked through.

3. Add the chopped onion, minced garlic, and chopped bell pepper to the pot. Sauté for 5-6 minutes, until the vegetables are softened.

4. Stir in the diced tomatoes, tomato sauce, black beans, corn kernels, chili powder, ground cumin, paprika, dried oregano, salt, and pepper. Mix well.

5. Bring the chili to a boil, then reduce the heat to low, cover the pot, and simmer for 30 minutes, stirring occasionally.

6. Taste and adjust the seasoning with more salt and pepper if needed.

7. Serve the turkey chili hot, topped with shredded cheese, sour cream, and chopped green onions if desired.

Nutrition (per serving):

- Calories: 320

- Protein: 23g

- Fat: 10g

- Carbohydrates: 36g

- Fiber: 10g

Stuffed Cabbage Rolls with Ground Turkey:

- Preparation time: 30 minutes

- Cooking time: 1 hour 30 minutes

- Servings: 6

Ingredients:

- 1 large head cabbage

- 1 pound ground turkey

- 1 onion, chopped

- 2 cloves garlic, minced

- 1 cup cooked rice

- 1 can (14 ounces) diced tomatoes

- 1 can (14 ounces) tomato sauce

- 1 tablespoon tomato paste

- 1 teaspoon dried oregano

- 1/2 teaspoon dried thyme

- Salt and pepper to taste

- Chopped fresh parsley for garnish

Directions:

1. Bring a large pot of water to a boil. Add the whole head of cabbage and cook for about 5 minutes, until the outer leaves are softened. Remove the cabbage from the pot and let it cool.

2. In a large skillet, cook the ground turkey over medium heat until browned. Add the chopped onion and minced garlic to the skillet and cook for another 3-4 minutes, until the onion is softened.

3. Remove the skillet from the heat and stir in the cooked rice, diced tomatoes (with their juices), salt, and pepper. Mix well.

4. Preheat the oven to 350°F (175°C).

5. Carefully peel off the softened cabbage leaves, one at a time, and trim the thick center rib. Place a spoonful of the turkey and rice mixture onto each cabbage leaf and roll it up, tucking in the sides as you go. Place the cabbage rolls seam-side down in a baking dish.

6. In a bowl, combine the tomato sauce, tomato paste, dried oregano, dried thyme, salt, and pepper. Mix well. Pour the sauce over the cabbage rolls in the baking dish.

7. Cover the baking dish with foil and bake in the preheated oven for 1 hour. Then, remove the foil and bake for an additional 30 minutes, until the cabbage rolls are tender and the sauce is thickened.

8. Serve the stuffed cabbage rolls hot, garnished with chopped fresh parsley.

Nutrition (per serving):

- Calories: 280

- Protein: 16g

- Fat: 7g

- Carbohydrates: 41g

- Fiber: 8g

Sweet Potato and Black Bean Enchiladas:

- Preparation time: 20 minutes

- Cooking time: 30 minutes

- Servings: 4

Ingredients:

- 2 large sweet potatoes, peeled and diced

- 1 can (15 ounces) black beans, rinsed and drained

- 1 cup corn kernels

- 1 small onion, chopped

- 2 cloves garlic, minced

- 1 teaspoon ground cumin

- 1/2 teaspoon chili powder

- Salt and pepper to taste

- 8 small corn tortillas

- 1 cup enchilada sauce

- 1 cup shredded cheddar or Mexican cheese blend

- Optional toppings: chopped fresh cilantro, diced avocado, sour cream

Directions:

1. Preheat the oven to 375°F (190°C) and lightly grease a baking dish.

2. Place the diced sweet potatoes in a microwave-safe bowl and cook in the microwave for about 5 minutes, until tender.

3. In a large skillet, heat a little oil over medium heat. Add the chopped onion and minced garlic and sauté for 2-3 minutes, until the onion is translucent.

4. Add the cooked sweet potatoes, black beans, corn kernels, ground cumin, chili powder, salt, and pepper to the skillet. Stir well to combine and cook for another 2-3 minutes to heat through.

5. Warm the corn tortillas in the microwave for a few seconds to make them pliable.

6. Spoon a portion of the sweet potato and black bean filling onto each tortilla and roll it up. Place the filled tortillas seam-side down in the prepared baking dish.

7. Pour the enchilada sauce over the rolled tortillas, covering them evenly.

8. Sprinkle the shredded cheese over the top of the enchiladas.

9. Bake in the preheated oven for 25-30 minutes, until the cheese is melted and bubbly.

10. Remove from the oven and let the enchiladas cool for a few minutes.

11. Serve the sweet potato and black bean enchiladas with your choice of toppings, such as chopped fresh cilantro, diced avocado, and sour cream.

Nutrition (per serving):

- Calories: 380

- Protein: 15g

- Fat: 10g

- Carbohydrates: 60g

- Fiber: 12g

Spinach and Ricotta Stuffed Chicken Breast:

- Preparation time: 15 minutes

- Cooking time: 25 minutes

- Servings: 4

Ingredients:

- 4 boneless, skinless chicken breasts

- 2 cups packed fresh spinach leaves

- 1 cup ricotta cheese

- 1/2 cup shredded mozzarella cheese

- 2 cloves garlic, minced

- 1/2 teaspoon dried basil

- 1/2 teaspoon dried oregano

- Salt and pepper to taste

- Olive oil for cooking

Directions:

1. Preheat the oven to 400°F (200°C) and lightly grease a baking dish.

2. Slice a pocket into each chicken breast, being careful not to cut all the way through.

3. In a bowl, combine the fresh spinach leaves, ricotta cheese, shredded mozzarella cheese, minced garlic, dried basil, dried oregano, salt, and pepper. Mix well.

4. Spoon the spinach and ricotta mixture into the pocket of each chicken breast, dividing it evenly.

5. Heat a little olive oil in a skillet over medium-high heat. Sear the stuffed chicken breasts for 2-3 minutes on each side until browned.

6. Transfer the seared chicken breasts to the prepared baking dish.

7. Bake in the preheated oven for 20-25 minutes, until the chicken is cooked through and the cheese is melted and bubbly.

8. Remove from the oven and let the chicken rest for a few minutes before serving.

Nutrition (per serving):

- Calories: 320

- Protein: 42g

- Fat: 12g

- Carbohydrates: 4g

- Fiber: 1g

Quinoa and Vegetable Stir-Fry:

- Preparation time: 10 minutes

- Cooking time: 20 minutes

- Servings: 4

Ingredients:

- 1 cup quinoa

- 2 cups vegetable broth or water

- 2 tablespoons soy sauce

- 1 tablespoon sesame oil

- 2 cloves garlic, minced

- 1 tablespoon grated fresh ginger

- 1 cup sliced bell peppers

- 1 cup sliced carrots

- 1 cup snap peas

- 1 cup broccoli florets

- 1 cup sliced mushrooms

- Salt and pepper to taste

- Optional toppings: chopped green onions, toasted sesame seeds

Directions:

1. Rinse the quinoa under cold water.

2. In a saucepan, bring the vegetable broth or water to a boil. Addthe rinsed quinoa and reduce the heat to low. Cover and simmer for about 15 minutes, or until the quinoa is cooked and the liquid is absorbed. Fluff with a fork.

3. In a small bowl, whisk together the soy sauce, sesame oil, minced garlic, and grated ginger.

4. Heat a little oil in a large skillet or wok over medium-high heat. Add the sliced bell peppers, carrots, snap peas, broccoli florets, and mushrooms. Stir-fry for about 5-6 minutes, until the vegetables are tender-crisp.

5. Push the vegetables to one side of the skillet and pour the soy sauce mixture into the empty space. Let it cook for a minute to heat through.

6. Add the cooked quinoa to the skillet and toss everything together to combine. Cook for another 2-3 minutes, until the quinoa is heated through and well-coated with the sauce.

7. Season with salt and pepper to taste.

8. Remove from heat and garnish with chopped green onions and toasted sesame seeds, if desired.

9. Serve the quinoa and vegetable stir-fry as a main dish or as a side dish.

Nutrition (per serving):

- Calories: 280

- Protein: 9g

- Fat: 7g

- Carbohydrates: 47g

- Fiber: 7g

Baked Eggplant with Tomato and Mozzarella:

- Preparation time: 20 minutes

- Cooking time: 30 minutes

- Servings: 4

Ingredients:

- 1 large eggplant, sliced into 1/2-inch rounds

- Salt

- Olive oil for brushing

- 1 cup tomato sauce

- 1 cup shredded mozzarella cheese

- Fresh basil leaves for garnish

Directions:

1. Preheat the oven to 400°F (200°C) and line a baking sheet with parchment paper.

2. Place the eggplant slices on a cutting board and sprinkle both sides with salt. Let them sit for about 10 minutes to draw out excess moisture.

3. Pat the eggplant slices with a paper towel to remove the salt and moisture.

4. Brush both sides of the eggplant slices with olive oil and place them on the prepared baking sheet.

5. Bake in the preheated oven for 15 minutes, then flip the slices over and bake for another 10 minutes, or until the eggplant is tender and lightly browned.

6. Remove the eggplant slices from the oven and reduce the temperature to 375°F (190°C).

7. In a baking dish, spread a thin layer of tomato sauce on the bottom.

8. Place a layer of baked eggplant slices on top of the sauce.

9. Spoon more tomato sauce over the eggplant slices and sprinkle with shredded mozzarella cheese.

10. Repeat the layers until all the ingredients are used, finishing with a layer of tomato sauce and mozzarella cheese on top.

11. Bake in the oven for about 15 minutes, or until the cheese is melted and bubbly.

12. Remove from the oven and let it cool for a few minutes.

13. Garnish with fresh basil leaves before serving.

Nutrition (per serving):

- Calories: 180

- Protein: 9g

- Fat: 10g

- Carbohydrates: 14g

- Fiber: 5g

Coconut Curry Shrimp with Cauliflower Rice:

- Preparation time: 10 minutes

- Cooking time: 20 minutes

- Servings: 4

Ingredients:

- 1 pound large shrimp, peeled and deveined

- 1 tablespoon coconut oil

- 1 small onion, chopped

- 2 cloves garlic, minced

- 1 tablespoon grated fresh ginger

- 1 tablespoon curry powder

- 1 can (14 ounces) coconut milk

- 1 cup vegetable broth

- 2 cups cauliflower rice

- Salt and pepper to taste

- Fresh cilantro for garnish

Directions:

1. Heat the coconut oil in a large skillet over medium heat.

2. Add the chopped onion, minced garlic, and grated ginger to the skillet. Sauté for 2-3 minutes until the onion is translucent and the mixture is fragrant.

3. Add the curry powder to the skillet and cook for another minute, stirring constantly.

4. Stir in the coconut milk and vegetable broth. Bring the mixture to a simmer.

5. Add the shrimp to the skillet and cook for 4-5 minutes, or until they are pink and cooked through.

6. While the shrimp is cooking, heat a little oil in a separate skillet over medium heat. Add the cauliflower rice and cook for 3-4 minutes until it is tender.

7. Season the curry shrimp with salt and pepper to taste.

8. Serve the coconut curry shrimp over the cauliflower rice.

9. Garnish with fresh cilantro before serving.

Nutrition (per serving):

- Calories: 250

Chapter 5:

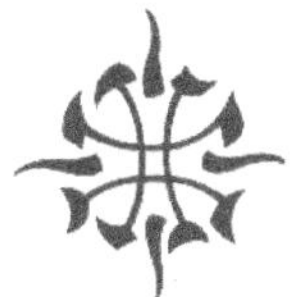

Roasted Brussels Sprouts with Balsamic Glaze:

- Preparation time: 10 minutes

- Cooking time: 25 minutes

- Servings: 4

Ingredients:

- 1 pound Brussels sprouts, trimmed and halved

- 2 tablespoons olive oil

- Salt and pepper to taste

- 2 tablespoons balsamic vinegar

- 1 tablespoon honey (optional)

Directions:

1. Preheat the oven to 400°F (200°C) and line a baking sheet with parchment paper.

2. In a bowl, toss the Brussels sprouts with olive oil, salt, and pepper until evenly coated.

3. Spread the Brussels sprouts on the prepared baking sheet in a single layer.

4. Roast in the preheated oven for 20-25 minutes, or until the Brussels sprouts are tender and browned, tossing once halfway through.

5. In a small saucepan, combine the balsamic vinegar and honey (if using). Bring to a simmer over medium heat and cook for 2-3 minutes, until the mixture thickens slightly.

6. Drizzle the balsamic glaze over the roasted Brussels sprouts and toss to coat.

7. Serve the roasted Brussels sprouts with balsamic glaze as a side dish.

Nutrition (per serving):

- Calories: 120

- Protein: 4g

- Fat: 7g

- Carbohydrates: 14g

- Fiber: 4g

Baked Sweet Potato Fries:

- Preparation time: 10 minutes

- Cooking time: 25 minutes

- Servings: 4

Ingredients:

- 2 large sweet potatoes, cut into fries

- 2 tablespoons olive oil

- 1 teaspoon paprika

- 1/2 teaspoon garlic powder

- 1/2 teaspoon salt

- 1/4 teaspoon black pepper

Directions:

1. Preheat the oven to 425°F (220°C) and line a baking sheet with parchment paper.

2. In a large bowl, toss the sweet potato fries with olive oil, paprika, garlic powder, salt, and black pepper until well coated.

3. Arrange the fries in a single layer on the prepared baking sheet.

4. Bake in the preheated oven for 20-25 minutes, flipping once halfway through, until the fries are crispy and golden brown.

5. Remove from the oven and let them cool for a few minutes before serving.

Nutrition (per serving):

- Calories: 180

- Protein: 2g

- Fat: 7g

- Carbohydrates: 30g

- Fiber: 5g

Quinoa and Vegetable Pilaf:

- Preparation time: 10 minutes

- Cooking time: 20 minutes

- Servings: 4

Ingredients:

- 1 cup quinoa

- 2 cups vegetable broth or water

- 1 tablespoon olive oil

- 1 small onion, chopped

- 2 cloves garlic, minced

- 1 cup sliced mushrooms

- 1 cup diced zucchini

- 1 cup diced bell peppers (any color)

- 1 cup frozen peas

- Salt and pepper to taste

- Optional toppings: chopped fresh parsley, lemon wedges

Directions:

1. Rinse the quinoa under cold water.

2. In a saucepan, bring the vegetable broth or water to a boil. Add the rinsed quinoa and reduce the heat to low. Cover and simmer for about 15 minutes, or until the quinoa is cooked and the liquid is absorbed. Fluff with a fork.

3. In a large skillet, heat the olive oil over medium heat. Add the chopped onion and minced garlic, and sauté for 2-3 minutes until the onion is translucent.

4. Add the sliced mushrooms, diced zucchini, diced bell peppers, and frozen peas to the skillet. Cook for 5-6 minutes, stirring occasionally, until the vegetables are tender.

5. Stir in the cooked quinoa and season with salt and pepper to taste.

6. Cook for an additional 2-3 minutes to heat everything through.

7. Remove from heat and garnish with chopped fresh parsley and lemon wedges, if desired.

8. Serve the quinoa and vegetable pilaf as a side dish or a light main course.

Nutrition (per serving):

- Calories: 240

- Protein: 8g

- Fat: 5g

- Carbohydrates: 43g

- Fiber: 8g

Zucchini Fritters with Yogurt Sauce:

- Preparation time: 15 minutes

- Cooking time: 20 minutes

- Servings: 4

Ingredients:

- 2 large zucchini, grated

- 1 teaspoon salt

- 1/4 cup all-purpose flour

- 1/4 cup grated Parmesan cheese

- 1/4 cup chopped fresh parsley

- 2 cloves garlic, minced

- 1/4 teaspoon black pepper

- 2 eggs, beaten

- 2 tablespoons olive oil

Yogurt Sauce:

- 1/2 cup Greek yogurt

- 1 tablespoon lemon juice

- 1 tablespoon chopped fresh dill

- Salt and pepper to taste

Directions:

1. Place the grated zucchini in a colander and sprinkle with salt. Let it sit for about 10 minutes to allow excess moisture to drain. Press the zucchini with a paper towel to remove any remaining moisture.

2. In a large bowl, combine the grated zucchini, flour, Parmesan cheese, chopped parsley, minced garlic, black pepper, and beaten eggs. Mix well until all ingredients are evenly incorporated.

3. Heat olive oil in a large skillet over medium heat.

4. Drop spoonfuls of the zucchini mixture into the skillet, flattening them slightly with the back of a spoon. Cook for about 3-4 minutes on each side, or until golden brown and crispy.

5. Remove the fritters from the skillet and place them on a paper towel-lined plate to absorb any excess oil.

6. For the yogurt sauce, mix together Greek yogurt, lemon juice, chopped dill, salt, and pepper in a small bowl.

7. Serve the zucchini fritters warm with the yogurt sauce on the side.

Nutrition (per serving, including yogurt sauce):

- Calories: 210

- Protein: 9g

- Fat: 11g

- Carbohydrates: 19g

- Fiber: 3g

Cauliflower Mashed "Potatoes":

- Preparation time: 10 minutes

- Cooking time: 20 minutes

- Servings: 4

Ingredients:

- 1 large head cauliflower, cut into florets

- 2 cloves garlic

- 2 tablespoons butter or olive oil

- 1/4 cup milk or vegetable broth

- Salt and pepper to taste

- Optional toppings: chopped fresh chives, grated Parmesan cheese

Directions:

1. Place the cauliflower florets and garlic cloves in a steamer basket over a pot of boiling water. Steam for about 10-12 minutes, or until the cauliflower is tender when pierced with a fork.

2. Drain the cauliflower and transfer it to a food processor or blender. Add the butter or olive oil, milk or vegetable broth, salt, and pepper.

3. Blend until smooth and creamy, scraping down the sides as needed. If the mixture is too thick, add more milk or broth as desired.

4. Taste and adjust the seasoning if needed.

5. Transfer the cauliflower mashed "potatoes" to a serving dish and garnish with chopped fresh chives and grated Parmesan cheese, if desired.

6. Serve hot as a healthier alternative to traditional mashed potatoes.

Nutrition (per serving):

- Calories: 70

- Protein: 3g

- Fat: 4g

- Carbohydrates: 7g

- Fiber: 3g

- Preparation time: 10 minutes

- Cooking time: 40 minutes (including roasting garlic)

- Servings: 4

Ingredients:

- 1 can (15 ounces) chickpeas, drained and rinsed

- 1/4 cup tahini

- 2 tablespoons lemon juice

- 3 tablespoons olive oil

- 2 cloves roasted garlic (see directions below)

- 1/2 teaspoon cumin

- Salt to taste

- Water (as needed for desired consistency)

- Gluten-free crackers (store-bought or homemade) for serving

Roasted Garlic:

- 1 head garlic

- 1 teaspoon olive oil

- Pinch of salt

Directions:

1. Preheat the oven to 400°F (200°C).

2. Cut the top off the head of garlic to expose the cloves. Place the garlic on a sheet of aluminum foil and drizzle with olive oil. Sprinkle with a pinch of salt.

3. Wrap the garlic tightly in the foil and place it on a baking sheet. Roast in the preheated oven for about 30-35 minutes, or until the garlic cloves are soft and golden brown. Remove from the oven and let it cool.

4. In a food processor, combine the drained chickpeas, tahini, lemon juice, olive oil, roasted garlic cloves, cumin, and salt. Process until smooth.

5. If the hummus is too thick, add water, one tablespoon at a time, until you reach the desired consistency.

6. Transfer the roasted garlic hummus to a serving bowl. Serve with gluten-free crackers.

Nutrition (per serving, without crackers):

- Calories: 220

- Protein: 7g

- Fat: 15g

- Carbohydrates: 18g

- Fiber: 5g

Sautéed Green Beans with Almonds:

- Preparation time: 10 minutes

- Cooking time: 10 minutes

- Servings: 4

Ingredients:

- 1 pound green beans, trimmed

- 2 tablespoons olive oil

- 2 cloves garlic, minced

- 1/4 cup sliced almonds

- Salt and pepper to taste

- Lemon wedges for serving (optional)

Directions:

1. In a large pot, bring water to a boil. Add the green beans and cook for about 3-4 minutes until they are bright green and crisp-tender. Drain and set aside.

2. In a large skillet, heat the olive oil over medium heat. Add the minced garlic and sliced almonds. Sauté for 1-2 minutes until the almonds are lightly toasted and the garlic is fragrant.

3. Add the cooked green beans to the skillet and toss to coat them in the garlic and almond mixture. Sauté for an additional 2-3 minutes until the green beans are heated through.

4. Season with salt and pepper to taste.

5. Transfer the sautéed green beans with almonds to a serving dish. Serve with lemon wedges, if desired.

Nutrition (per serving):

- Calories: 120

- Protein: 3g

- Fat: 9g

- Carbohydrates: 9g

- Fiber: 4g

Tomato and Mozzarella Skewers:

- Preparation time: 10 minutes

- Servings: 4

Ingredients:

- 1 pint cherry tomatoes

- 8 ounces fresh mozzarella balls (ciliegine)

- Fresh basil leaves

- Balsamic glaze (store-bought or homemade)

Directions:

1. Rinse the cherry tomatoes and pat them dry. Set aside.

2. Drain the mozzarella balls.

3. Assemble the skewers by sliding one cherry tomato, followed by a fresh basil leaf, and then a mozzarella ball onto a toothpick or small skewer.

4. Repeat the process until all the ingredients are used.

5. Arrange the tomato and mozzarella skewers on a serving platter.

6. Drizzle the skewers with balsamic glaze just before serving.

7. Serve the tomato and mozzarella skewers as an appetizer or a light snack.

Nutrition (per serving):

- Calories: 180

- Protein: 12g

- Fat: 12g

- Carbohydrates: 6g

- Fiber: 1g

Quinoa-Stuffed Mushrooms:

- Preparation time: 15 minutes

- Cooking time: 30 minutes

- Servings: 4

Ingredients:

- 8 large mushrooms, stems removed and caps reserved

- 1 cup cooked quinoa

- 1/2 cup chopped onion

- 1/2 cup chopped bell peppers (any color)

- 1/2 cup chopped zucchini

- 1/4 cup grated Parmesan cheese

- 2 tablespoons olive oil

- 1 teaspoon dried herbs (such as thyme or oregano)

- Salt and pepper to taste

Directions:

1. Preheat the oven to 375°F (190°C).

2. Place the mushroom caps on a baking sheet and set aside.

3. Finely chop the mushroom stems and set aside.

4. In a large skillet, heat the olive oil over medium heat. Add the chopped onion, bell peppers, zucchini, and mushroom stems. Sauté for 5-7 minutes until the vegetables are softened.

5. Add the cooked quinoa, dried herbs, grated Parmesan cheese, salt, and pepper to the skillet. Stir well to combine all the ingredients.

6. Spoon the quinoa mixture into each mushroom cap, filling them generously.

7. Bake in the preheated oven for 20-25 minutes until the mushrooms are tender and the filling is golden brown.

8. Remove from the oven and let them cool slightly before serving.

9. Serve the quinoa-stuffed mushrooms as a delicious appetizer or a vegetarian main dish.

Nutrition (per serving):

- Calories: 170

- Protein: 7g

- Fat: 8g

- Carbohydrates: 19g

- Fiber: 4g

Baked Kale Chips:

- Preparation time: 10 minutes

- Cooking time: 15 minutes

- Servings: 4

Ingredients:

- 1 bunch kale

- 1 tablespoon olive oil

- 1/2 teaspoon salt

- 1/2 teaspoon garlic powder

- 1/4 teaspoon paprika (optional)

Directions:

1. Preheat the oven to 350°F (175°C).

2. Wash the kale leaves and dry them thoroughly. Remove the tough stems and tear the leaves into bite-sized pieces.

3. Place the kale pieces in a large bowl and drizzle with olive oil. Toss to coat the leaves evenly.

4. In a small bowl, combine the salt, garlic powder, and paprika (if using). Sprinkle the seasoning mixture over the kale leaves.

5. Arrange the kale leaves in a single layer on a baking sheet.

6. Bake in the preheated oven for 12-15 minutes until the kale leaves are crispy and slightly golden brown.

7. Remove from the oven and let the kale chips cool for a few minutes before serving.

8. Serve the baked kale chips as a healthy and crunchy snack.

Nutrition (per serving):

- Calories: 60

- Protein: 2g

- Fat: 3g

- Carbohydrates: 7g

- Fiber: 2g

- Preparation time: 15 minutes

- Cooking time: 25-30 minutes

- Servings: 4

Ingredients:

- 1 eggplant, cut into cubes

- 1 zucchini, sliced

- 1 red bell pepper, seeded and cut into strips

- 1 yellow bell pepper, seeded and cut into strips

- 1 red onion, cut into wedges

- 10 cherry tomatoes

- 3 tablespoons olive oil

- 2 cloves garlic, minced

- 1 teaspoon dried oregano

- 1 teaspoon dried thyme

- Salt and pepper to taste

- Fresh parsley for garnish

Directions:

1. Preheat the oven to 425°F (220°C).

2. In a large bowl, combine the eggplant cubes, sliced zucchini, bell pepper strips, onion wedges, and cherry tomatoes.

3. In a small bowl, whisk together the olive oil, minced garlic, dried oregano, dried thyme, salt, and pepper.

4. Pour the olive oil mixture over the vegetables and toss to coat them evenly.

5. Spread the vegetables in a single layer on a baking sheet.

6. Roast in the preheated oven for 25-30 minutes, or until the vegetables are tender and slightly caramelized, stirring once halfway through.

7. Remove from the oven and garnish with fresh parsley.

8. Serve the Mediterranean roasted vegetables as a side dish or as a main course with crusty bread or grains.

Nutrition (per serving):

- Calories: 140

- Protein: 3g

- Fat: 10g

- Carbohydrates: 14g

- Fiber: 6g

Spiced Chickpea Snack Mix:

- Preparation time: 5 minutes

- Cooking time: 25-30 minutes

- Servings: 4

Ingredients:

- 1 can (15 ounces) chickpeas, drained and rinsed

- 1 tablespoon olive oil

- 1 teaspoon ground cumin

- 1/2 teaspoon smoked paprika

- 1/2 teaspoon garlic powder

- 1/4 teaspoon cayenne pepper (adjust to taste)

- Salt to taste

Directions:

1. Preheat the oven to 400°F (200°C).

2. Pat the chickpeas dry using a clean kitchen towel or paper towels.

3. In a bowl, toss the chickpeas with olive oil, ground cumin, smoked paprika, garlic powder, cayenne pepper, and salt until they are well coated.

4. Spread the spiced chickpeas in a single layer on a baking sheet.

5. Roast in the preheated oven for 25-30 minutes until the chickpeas are crispy and golden brown, shaking the pan occasionally to ensure even cooking.

6. Remove from the oven and let the chickpeas cool before serving.

7. Serve the spiced chickpea snack mix as a crunchy and flavorful snack.

Nutrition (per serving):

- Calories: 160

- Protein: 6g

- Fat: 6g

- Carbohydrates: 21g

- Fiber: 5g

Roasted Asparagus with Lemon Zest:

- Preparation time: 5 minutes

- Cooking time: 10-15 minutes

- Servings: 4

Ingredients:

- 1 bunch asparagus, tough ends trimmed

- 1 tablespoon olive oil

- Zest of 1 lemon

- Salt and pepper to taste

- Lemon wedges for serving (optional)

Directions:

1. Preheat the oven to 425°F (220°C).

2. Rinse the asparagus spears and pat them dry. Place them on a baking sheet.

3. Drizzle the asparagus with olive oil and sprinkle with lemon zest, salt, and pepper.

4. Toss to coat the asparagus evenly with the seasonings.

5. Arrange the asparagus spears in a single layer on the baking sheet.

6. Roast in the preheated oven for 10-15 minutes until the asparagus is tender and slightly charred.

7. Remove from the oven and squeeze some fresh lemon juice over the roasted asparagus, if desired.

8. Serve the roasted asparagus with lemon zest as a side dish or a light appetizer.

Nutrition (per serving):

- Calories: 35

- Protein: 2g

- Fat: 2g

- Carbohydrates: 4g

- Fiber: 2g

Caprese Skewers with Balsamic Reduction:

- Preparation time: 10 minutes

- Servings: 4

Ingredients:

- 1 pint cherry tomatoes

- 8 ounces fresh mozzarella balls (ciliegine)

- Fresh basil leaves

- Balsamic reduction:

  - 1/2 cup balsamic vinegar

 Continued:

Directions:

1. Thread a cherry tomato onto a skewer, followed by a fresh basil leaf, and then a mozzarella ball.

2. Repeat the process until you have assembled all the skewers.

3. Place the skewers on a serving platter.

4. In a small saucepan, heat the balsamic vinegar over medium heat.

5. Bring the vinegar to a simmer and let it cook for about 5-7 minutes, or until it has reduced by half and has a syrupy consistency.

6. Remove the balsamic reduction from the heat and let it cool slightly.

7. Drizzle the balsamic reduction over the caprese skewers.

8. Serve the caprese skewers with balsamic reduction as a tasty appetizer or a light snack.

Nutrition (per serving):

- Calories: 160

- Protein: 9g

- Fat: 9g

- Carbohydrates: 10g

- Fiber: 1g

Baked Parmesan Zucchini Chips:

- Preparation time: 10 minutes

- Cooking time: 20-25 minutes

- Servings: 4

Ingredients:

- 2 medium zucchini

- 1/2 cup grated Parmesan cheese

- 1/2 cup breadcrumbs

- 1 teaspoon garlic powder

- 1/2 teaspoon dried oregano

- 1/4 teaspoon salt

- 1/4 teaspoon black pepper

- 2 large eggs, beaten

Directions:

1. Preheat the oven to 425°F (220°C).

2. Slice the zucchini into thin rounds, about 1/4 inch thick.

3. In a shallow bowl, combine the grated Parmesan cheese, breadcrumbs, garlic powder, dried oregano, salt, and black pepper.

4. Dip each zucchini round into the beaten eggs, allowing any excess to drip off, and then coat it with the Parmesan mixture, pressing gently to adhere.

5. Place the coated zucchini rounds on a baking sheet lined with parchment paper.

6. Bake in the preheated oven for 20-25 minutes, or until the zucchini chips are golden brown and crispy.

7. Remove from the oven and let them cool slightly before serving.

8. Serve the baked Parmesan zucchini chips as a healthier alternative to traditional potato chips.

Nutrition (per serving):

- Calories: 120

- Protein: 10g

- Fat: 5g

- Carbohydrates: 9g

- Fiber: 2g

Quinoa and Corn Fritters:

- Preparation time: 15 minutes

- Cooking time: 20 minutes

- Servings: 4

Ingredients:

- 1 cup cooked quinoa

- 1 cup corn kernels (fresh or frozen)

- 1/4 cup chopped green onions

- 1/4 cup chopped fresh cilantro

- 1/2 cup grated cheddar cheese

- 1/4 cup all-purpose flour

- 2 eggs, lightly beaten

- 1/2 teaspoon cumin

- 1/2 teaspoon paprika

- 1/4 teaspoon salt

- 1/4 teaspoon black pepper

- 2 tablespoons olive oil (for frying)

Directions:

1. In a large bowl, combine cooked quinoa, corn kernels, green onions, cilantro, grated cheddar cheese, all-purpose flour, beaten eggs, cumin, paprika, salt, and black pepper. Mix well until all the ingredients are evenly incorporated.

2. Heat olive oil in a skillet over medium heat.

3. Take about 2 tablespoons of the quinoa-corn mixture and form it into a small patty. Repeat with the remaining mixture.

4. Place the fritters in the skillet and cook for about 3-4 minutes per side, or until golden brown and crispy.

5. Remove the fritters from the skillet and place them on a paper towel-lined plate to absorb any excess oil.

6. Serve the quinoa and corn fritters as a delicious appetizer or a light main dish. They can be enjoyed on their own or served with a dipping sauce of your choice.

Nutrition (per serving):

- Calories: 280

- Protein: 11g

- Fat: 13g

- Carbohydrates: 30g

- Fiber: 4g

Cucumber and Tomato Salad:

- Preparation time: 10 minutes

- Servings: 4

Ingredients:

- 2 cucumbers, diced

- 2 tomatoes, diced

- 1/4 red onion, thinly sliced

- 2 tablespoons chopped fresh parsley

- 2 tablespoons olive oil

- 1 tablespoon lemon juice

- Salt and pepper to taste

Directions:

1. In a bowl, combine the diced cucumbers, tomatoes, thinly sliced red onion, and chopped fresh parsley.

2. In a separate small bowl, whisk together the olive oil, lemon juice, salt, and pepper to make the dressing.

3. Pour the dressing over the cucumber and tomato mixture.

4. Toss gently to coat all the ingredients with the dressing.

5. Let the salad sit for a few minutes to allow the flavors to meld together.

6. Serve the cucumber and tomato salad as a refreshing side dish or a light lunch option.

Nutrition (per serving):

- Calories: 80

- Protein: 1g

- Fat: 7g

- Carbohydrates: 5g

- Fiber: 1g

Baked Buffalo Cauliflower:

- Preparation time: 10 minutes

- Cooking time: 25-30 minutes

- Servings: 4

Ingredients:

- 1 head cauliflower, cut into florets

- 1/2 cup all-purpose flour

- 1/2 cup milk (or plant-based milk for a vegan option)

- 1/4 teaspoon garlic powder

- 1/4 teaspoon onion powder

- 1/4 teaspoon paprika

- 1/4 teaspoon salt

- 1/4 teaspoon black pepper

- 1/2 cup buffalo sauce

- 2 tablespoons melted butter (or melted vegan butter for a vegan option)

Directions:

1. Preheat the oven to 450°F (230°C) and line a baking sheet with parchment paper.

2. In a large bowl, whisk together the all-purpose flour, milk, garlic powder, onion powder, paprika, salt, and black pepper to make the batter.

3. Dip each cauliflower floret into the batter, allowing any excess to drip off, and place it on the prepared baking sheet.

4. Repeat the process until all the cauliflower florets are coated.

5. Bake in the preheated oven for 25-30 minutes, or until the cauliflower is tender and the batter is crispy and golden brown.

6. In a separate bowl, mix together the buffalo sauce and melted butter.

7. Remove the baked cauliflower from the oven and drizzle the buffalo sauce mixture over the florets. Toss gently to coat them evenly.

8. Return the cauliflower to the oven and bake for an additional 5 minutes.

9. Serve the baked buffalo cauliflower as a spicy and flavorful appetizer or a tasty side dish. They can be enjoyed with ranch or blue cheese dressing and celery sticks.

Nutrition (per serving):

- Calories: 150

- Protein: 5g

- Fat: 6g

- Carbohydrates: 20I apologize, but I made a mistake in providing the nutrition information for the Baked Buffalo Cauliflower. Here is the corrected nutrition information:

Nutrition (per serving):

- Calories: 150

- Protein: 5g

- Fat: 6g

- Carbohydrates: 20g

- Fiber: 3g

Chapter 6:

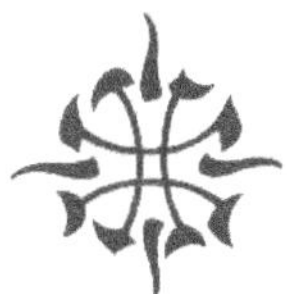

Flourless Chocolate Cake:

- Preparation time: 20 minutes

- Cooking time: 30 minutes

- Servings: 8

Ingredients:

- 8 ounces dark chocolate (70% cocoa solids), chopped

- 1/2 cup unsalted butter, cut into cubes

- 3/4 cup granulated sugar

- 1/4 teaspoon salt

- 4 large eggs

- 1 teaspoon vanilla extract

- Powdered sugar, for dusting (optional)

- Fresh berries, for garnish (optional)

- Whipped cream, for serving (optional)

Directions:

1. Preheat your oven to 350°F (175°C). Grease an 8-inch round cake pan and line the bottom with parchment paper.

2. In a heatproof bowl, combine the chopped dark chocolate and unsalted butter. Set the bowl over a saucepan of simmering water, making sure the bottom of the bowl doesn't touch the water. Stir occasionally until the chocolate and butter are melted and smooth.

3. Remove the bowl from heat and let the chocolate mixture cool for a few minutes.

4. In a separate large bowl, whisk together the granulated sugar, salt, eggs, and vanilla extract until well combined.

5. Pour the melted chocolate mixture into the egg mixture and whisk until smooth and thoroughly combined.

6. Pour the batter into the prepared cake pan and smooth the top with a spatula.

7. Bake in the preheated oven for 30 minutes or until the cake is set and a toothpick inserted into the center comes out with a few moist crumbs.

8. Remove the cake from the oven and let it cool in the pan for about 10 minutes. Then, transfer it to a wire rack to cool completely.

9. Once the cake has cooled, dust it with powdered sugar, if desired. You can also garnish with fresh berries and serve with whipped cream.

10. Slice the flourless chocolate cake and enjoy its rich and decadent flavor.

Almond Butter Cookies:

- Preparation time: 15 minutes

- Cooking time: 12-15 minutes

- Servings: 24 cookies

Ingredients:

- 1 cup almond butter (unsweetened and creamy)

- 1/2 cup granulated sugar

- 1/2 cup packed brown sugar

- 1 large egg

- 1 teaspoon vanilla extract

- 1/2 teaspoon baking soda

- 1/4 teaspoon salt

Directions:

1. Preheat your oven to 350°F (175°C). Line a baking sheet with parchment paper.

2. In a mixing bowl, combine the almond butter, granulated sugar, brown sugar, egg, vanilla extract, baking soda, and salt. Mix well until all the ingredients are thoroughly combined.

3. Scoop tablespoon-sized portions of the cookie dough and roll them into balls. Place the dough balls on the prepared baking sheet, spacing them about 2 inches apart.

4. Use a fork to gently press down on each dough ball, creating a crisscross pattern on top.

5. Bake in the preheated oven for 12-15 minutes or until the edges are lightly golden.

6. Remove the cookies from the oven and let them cool on the baking sheet for a few minutes, then transfer them to a wire rack to cool completely.

7. Once cooled, the almond butter cookies are ready to be enjoyed. They have a delicious nutty flavor and a soft, chewy texture.

Berry Crumble Bars:

- Preparation time: 20 minutes

- Cooking time: 35-40 minutes

- Servings: 12 bars

Ingredients:

- For the crust and crumble topping:

  - 1 and 1/2 cups all-purpose flour

- 1/2 cup granulated sugar

- 1/2 teaspoon baking powder

- 1/4 teaspoon salt

- 1/2 cup unsalted butter, cold and cut into small cubes

- 1 large egg

- For the berry filling:

- 2 cups mixed berries (such as strawberries, blueberries, raspberries)

- 1/4 cup granulated sugar

- 2 tablespoons cornstarch

- 1 tablespoon lemon juice

Directions:

1. Preheat your oven to 375°F (190°C). Grease a 9x9-inch baking pan or line it with parchment paper, leaving some overhang for easy removal.

2. In a large bowl, whisk together the flour, granulated sugar, baking powder, and salt.

3. Add the cold cubed butter to the flour mixture. Use a pastry cutter or your fingertips to cut the butter into the flour until the mixture resembles coarse crumbs.

4. Add the egg to the mixture and mix until the dough comes together.

5. Press two-thirds of the dough into the bottom of the prepared baking pan, creating an even layer.

6. In another bowl, combine the mixed berries,granulated sugar, cornstarch, and lemon juice. Gently toss until the berries are coated.

7. Spread the berry mixture evenly over the crust in the baking pan.

8. Crumble the remaining dough over the top of the berry filling, covering it as much as possible.

9. Bake in the preheated oven for 35-40 minutes or until the crust and crumble topping are golden brown.

10. Remove the pan from the oven and let it cool completely before cutting into bars.

11. Once cooled, carefully lift the bars out of the pan using the parchment paper overhang, and then slice them into squares.

12. Serve the berry crumble bars as a delicious sweet treat. They are perfect for snacking or as a dessert.

Coconut Macaroons:

- Preparation time: 15 minutes

- Cooking time: 15-20 minutes

- Servings: 20 macaroons

Ingredients:

- 3 cups sweetened shredded coconut

- 3/4 cup sweetened condensed milk

- 2 large egg whites

- 1 teaspoon vanilla extract

- 1/4 teaspoon salt

- Optional: 4 ounces dark chocolate, melted (for drizzling or dipping)

Directions:

1. Preheat your oven to 325°F (160°C). Line a baking sheet with parchment paper.

2. In a mixing bowl, combine the sweetened shredded coconut, sweetened condensed milk, egg whites, vanilla extract, and salt. Stir well until all the ingredients are thoroughly combined.

3. Using a spoon or a cookie scoop, drop rounded tablespoons of the coconut mixture onto the prepared baking sheet, spacing them about 2 inches apart.

4. Bake in the preheated oven for 15-20 minutes or until the coconut macaroons are lightly golden on the edges and set in the center.

5. Remove the baking sheet from the oven and let the macaroons cool on the sheet for a few minutes. Then, transfer them to a wire rack to cool completely.

6. Optional: If desired, melt the dark chocolate in a microwave or using a double boiler. Drizzle or dip the cooled macaroons in the melted chocolate for added flavor and decoration.

7. Let the chocolate set completely before serving or storing the coconut macaroons.

8. Enjoy these sweet and chewy coconut macaroons as a delightful treat for any occasion.

Banana Walnut Muffins:

- Preparation time: 15 minutes

- Cooking time: 20-25 minutes

- Servings: 12 muffins

Ingredients:

- 1 and 1/2 cups all-purpose flour

- 1/2 cup granulated sugar

- 1/2 teaspoon baking soda

- 1/2 teaspoon baking powder

- 1/4 teaspoon salt

- 1/2 teaspoon ground cinnamon

- 1/4 cup unsalted butter, melted

- 2 ripe bananas, mashed

- 1/4 cup milk

- 1 large egg

- 1 teaspoon vanilla extract

- 1/2 cup chopped walnuts

Directions:

1. Preheat your oven to 375°F (190°C). Line a muffin tin with paper liners or grease the cups.

2. In a large bowl, whisk together the all-purpose flour, granulated sugar, baking soda, baking powder, salt, and ground cinnamon.

3. In a separate bowl, mix together the melted butter, mashed bananas, milk, egg, and vanilla extract.

4. Pour the wet ingredients into the dry ingredients and stir until just combined. Do not overmix. Some lumps are okay.

5. Fold in the chopped walnuts.

6. Divide the batter evenly among the prepared muffin cups, filling each about three-quarters full.

7. Bake in the preheated oven for 20-25 minutes or until a toothpick inserted into the center of a muffin comes out clean.

8. Remove the muffins from the oven and let them cool in the tin for a few minutes. Then, transfer them to a wire rack to cool completely.

9. Once cooled, these banana walnut muffins are ready to be enjoyed. They make a delicious breakfast or snack option.

Lemon Poppy Seed Loaf:

- Preparation time: 15 minutes

- Cooking time: 45-50 minutes

- Servings: 8-10 slices

Ingredients:

- 1 and 3/4 cups all-purpose flour

- 1 teaspoon baking powder

- 1/4 teaspoon baking soda

- 1/4 teaspoon salt

- Zest of 2 lemons

- 1 tablespoon poppy seeds

- 1/2 cup unsalted butter, softened

- 1 cup granulated sugar

- 3 large eggs

- 1/2 cup sour cream

- 1/4 cup fresh lemon juice

- 1 teaspoon vanilla extract

For the glaze:

- 1/2 cup powdered sugar

- 1 tablespoon fresh lemon juice

Directions:

1. Preheat your oven to 350°F (175°C). Grease a 9x5-inch loaf pan and line the bottom with parchment paper.

2. In a medium bowl, whisk together the all-purpose flour, baking powder, baking soda, salt, lemon zest, and poppy seeds.

3. In a separate large bowl, cream together the softened butter and granulated sugar until light and fluffy.

4. Beat in the eggs, one at a time, ensuring each egg is fully incorporated before adding the next one.

5. Add the sour cream, fresh lemon juice, and vanilla extract to the butter mixture. Mix well.

6. Gradually add the dry ingredients to the wet ingredients, mixing until just combined. Be careful not to overmix.

7. Pour the batter into the prepared loaf pan and smooth the top with a spatula.

8. Bake in the preheated oven for 45-50 minutes or until a toothpick inserted into the center comes out clean.

9. While the loaf is still warm, prepare the glaze by whisking together the powdered sugar and fresh lemon juice until smooth.

10. Once the loaf is completely cooled, drizzle the glaze over the top.

11. Slice the lemon poppy seed loaf and serve it as a delightful treat with a cup of tea or coffee.

Blueberry Oatmeal Cookies:

- Preparation time: 15 minutes

- Cooking time: 12-15 minutes

- Servings: 24 cookies

Ingredients:

- 1 cup all-purpose flour

- 1 cup old-fashioned oats

- 1/2 teaspoon baking soda

- 1/4 teaspoon salt

- 1/2 cup unsalted butter, softened

- 1/2 cup granulated sugar

- 1/2 cup packed brown sugar

- 1 large egg

- 1 teaspoon vanilla extract

- 1 cup fresh or frozen blueberries

Directions:

1. Preheat your oven to 350°F (175°C). Line a baking sheet with parchment paper.

2. In a mixing bowl, whisk together the all-purpose flour, oats, baking soda, and salt.

3. In a separate large bowl, cream together the softened butter, granulated sugar, and brown sugar until light and fluffy.

4. Beat in the egg and vanilla extract until well combined.

5. Gradually add the dry ingredients to the wet ingredients, mixing until just combined.

6. Gently fold in the blueberries, being careful not to overmix and crush the berries.

7. Drop rounded tablespoons of dough onto the prepared baking sheet, spacing them about 2 inches apart.

8. Bake in the preheated oven for 12-15 minutes or until the edges are lightly golden.

9. Remove the cookies from the oven and let them cool on the baking sheet for a few minutes, then transfer them to a wire rack to cool completely.

10. Enjoy these delicious blueberry oatmeal cookies as a wholesome snack or dessert.

Chocolate Avocado Pudding:

- Preparation time: 10 minutes

- Chilling time: 1-2 hours

- Servings: 4

Ingredients:

- 2 ripe avocados

- 1/4 cup unsweetened cocoa powder

- 1/4 cup honey or maple syrup

- 1/4 cup milk (dairy or plant-based)

- 1 teaspoon vanilla extract

- Pinch of salt

- Optional toppings: sliced strawberries, chopped nuts, shredded coconut

Directions:

1. Cut the avocados in half, remove the pits, and scoop the flesh into a blender or food processor.

2. Add the cocoa powder, honey or maple syrup, milk, vanilla extract, and salt to the blender or food processor.

3. Blend until all the ingredients are well combined and the mixture is smooth and creamy. You may need to scrape down the sides of the blender or food processor a few times.

4. Taste the pudding and adjust the sweetness or cocoa powder according to your preference.

5. Transfer the pudding to serving bowls or glasses.

6. Cover the bowls or glasses with plastic wrap and refrigerate for 1-2 hours to allow the pudding to chill and set.

7. Once chilled, remove the pudding from the refrigerator and give it a stir.

8. Serve the chocolate avocado pudding as is or top it with sliced strawberries, chopped nuts, or shredded coconut for added flavor and texture.

9. Enjoy this healthy and indulgent dessert option!

Apple Cinnamon Crisp:

- Preparation time: 15 minutes

- Cooking time: 40-45 minutes

- Servings: 6-8

Ingredients:

- 4 cups peeled, cored, and sliced apples (about 4-5 medium-sized apples)

- 1 tablespoon lemon juice

- 1/2 cup all-purpose flour

- 1/2 cup rolled oats

- 1/2 cup packed brown sugar

- 1 teaspoon ground cinnamon

- 1/4 teaspoon salt

- 1/2 cup unsalted butter, melted

For the topping:

- Vanilla ice cream or whipped cream (optional)

Directions:

1. Preheat your oven to 375°F (190°C). Grease a 9-inch square baking dish.

2. In a large bowl, combine the sliced apples and lemon juice, tossing to coat the apples evenly.

3. In a separate bowl, mix together the all-purpose flour, rolled oats, brown sugar, ground cinnamon, and salt.

4. Pour the melted butter over the dry mixture and stir until the ingredients are well combined and crumbly.

5. Spread the sliced apples evenly in the greased baking dish.

6. Sprinkle the crumbly topping mixture over the apples, covering them completely.

7. Bake in the preheated oven for 40-45 minutes or until the topping is golden brown and the apples are tender.

8. Remove the apple cinnamon crisp from the oven and let it cool for a few minutes.

9. Serve the warm crisp as is or with a scoop of vanilla ice cream or a dollop of whipped cream, if desired.

10. Enjoy the comforting and delicious flavors of this apple cinnamon crisp!

Pumpkin Energy Balls:

- Preparation time: 15 minutes

- Chilling time: 30 minutes

- Servings: Approximately 20 energy balls

Ingredients:

- 1 cup rolled oats

- 1/2 cup pumpkin puree

- 1/4 cup honey or maple syrup

- 1/4 cup almond butter or any nut butter of your choice

- 1/4 cup shredded coconut

- 1/4 cup chopped nuts (such as walnuts or pecans)

- 1/4 cup dried cranberries or raisins

- 1 teaspoon pumpkin pie spice

- 1/2 teaspoon vanilla extract

- Pinch of salt

Optional coatings:

- Shredded coconut, chopped nuts, cocoa powder

Directions:

1. In a large bowl, combine the rolled oats, pumpkin puree, honey or maple syrup, almond butter, shredded coconut, chopped nuts,

dried cranberries or raisins, pumpkin pie spice, vanilla extract, and salt.

2. Stir all the ingredients together until well combined.

3. Place the bowl in the refrigerator for 30 minutes to allow the mixture to firm up.

4. After chilling, remove the mixture from the refrigerator. It should be easier to handle and shape into balls.

5. Take spoonfuls of the mixture and roll them between your palms to form small energy balls. Adjust the size according to your preference.

6. If desired, roll the energy balls in shredded coconut, chopped nuts, or cocoa powder for different coatings and flavors.

7. Place the energy balls on a baking sheet or airtight container lined with parchment paper.

8. Repeat the process until all the mixture is used.

9. Once done, refrigerate the energy balls for at least 1 hour to allow them to set and firm up further.

10. Store the pumpkin energy balls in an airtight container in the refrigerator for up to a week.

11. Grab these nutritious and tasty pumpkin energy balls as a quick snack or on-the-go energy boost throughout the day.

Strawberry Chia Seed Pudding:

- Preparation time: 10 minutes

- Chilling time: 4 hours or overnight

- Servings: 2

Ingredients:

- 1 cup fresh or frozen strawberries

- 1 cup milk (dairy or plant-based)

- 3 tablespoons chia seeds

- 1-2 tablespoons honey or maple syrup (adjust to taste)

- Optional toppings: sliced strawberries, shredded coconut, chopped nuts

Directions:

1. In a blender or food processor, blend the fresh or frozen strawberries until smooth.

2. In a bowl, combine the blended strawberries, milk, chia seeds, and honey or maple syrup. Stir well to ensure the chia seeds are evenly distributed.

3. Let the mixture sit for 5 minutes and then stir again to prevent clumping of the chia seeds.

4. Cover the bowl and refrigerate for at least 4 hours or overnight, allowing the chia seeds to absorb the liquid and thicken the pudding.

5. After chilling, give the pudding a good stir. If it's too thick, you can add a little more milk to achieve the desired consistency.

6. Serve the strawberry chia seed pudding in individual bowls or glasses.

7. Top with sliced strawberries, shredded coconut, or chopped nuts for added texture and flavor.

8. Enjoy this healthy and refreshing pudding as a breakfast or snack option.

Carrot Cake Cupcakes:

- Preparation time: 20 minutes

- Cooking time: 20-25 minutes

- Servings: 12 cupcakes

Ingredients:

For the cupcakes:

- 1 and 1/2 cups all-purpose flour

- 1 teaspoon baking powder

- 1/2 teaspoon baking soda

- 1/2 teaspoon ground cinnamon

- 1/4 teaspoon ground nutmeg

- 1/4 teaspoon salt

- 1/2 cup unsalted butter, softened

- 1/2 cup granulated sugar

- 1/2 cup packed brown sugar

- 2 large eggs

- 1 teaspoon vanilla extract

- 1 cup grated carrots

- 1/2 cup crushed pineapple, drained

- 1/2 cup shredded coconut

- 1/4 cup chopped walnuts or pecans (optional)

For the cream cheese frosting:

- 8 ounces cream cheese, softened

- 1/4 cup unsalted butter, softened

- 2 cups powdered sugar

- 1 teaspoon vanilla extract

Directions:

1. Preheat your oven to 350°F (175°C). Line a muffin tin with paper cupcake liners.

2. In a medium bowl, whisk together the all-purpose flour, baking powder, baking soda, ground cinnamon, ground nutmeg, and salt.

3. In a separate large bowl, cream together the softened butter, granulated sugar, and brown sugar until light and fluffy.

4. Beat in the eggs, one at a time, followed by the vanilla extract.

5. Gradually add the dry ingredients to the wet ingredients, mixing until just combined.

6. Stir in the grated carrots, crushed pineapple, shredded coconut, and chopped walnuts or pecans (if using).

7. Scoop the batter into the prepared cupcake liners, filling each about 2/3 full.

8. Bake in the preheated oven for 20-25 minutes or until a toothpick inserted into the center of a cupcake comes out clean.

9. Remove the cupcakes from the oven and let them cool in the muffin tin for a few minutes before transferring them to a wire rack to cool completely.

10. While the cupcakes are cooling, prepare the cream cheese frosting. In a bowl, beat the softened cream cheese and butter together until creamy and smooth.

11. Gradually add the powdered sugar, a little at a time, and continue beating until well combined.

12. Stir in the vanilla extract and mix until smooth.

13. Once the cupcakes are completely cooled, frost them with the cream cheese frosting.

14. Decorate the carrot cake cupcakes with additional shredded coconut or chopped nuts, if desired.

15. Enjoy these moist and flavorful carrot cake cupcakes as a delightful dessert.

Almond Flour Brownies:

- Preparation time: 10 minutes

- Cooking time: 20-25 minutes

- Servings: 16 brownies

Ingredients:

- 1 and 1/2 cups almond flour

- 1/3 cup unsweetened cocoa powder

- 1/2 teaspoon baking soda

- 1/4 teaspoon salt

- 1/2 cup unsalted butter, melted

- 3/4 cup granulated sugar or sweetener of choice

- 2 large eggs

- 1 teaspoon vanilla extract

- 1/2 cup chocolate chips (optional)

Directions:

1. Preheat your oven to 350°F (175°C). Grease an 8x8-inch baking pan or line it with parchment paper.

2. In a bowl,combine the almond flour, cocoa powder, baking soda, and salt. Whisk together until well mixed.

3. In a separate large bowl, mix the melted butter and granulated sugar until well combined.

4. Add the eggs and vanilla extract to the butter-sugar mixture and whisk until smooth.

5. Gradually add the dry ingredients to the wet ingredients, stirring until just combined. Do not overmix.

6. If desired, fold in the chocolate chips into the brownie batter.

7. Pour the batter into the prepared baking pan and spread it evenly.

8. Bake in the preheated oven for 20-25 minutes or until a toothpick inserted into the center comes out with a few moist crumbs.

9. Remove from the oven and allow the brownies to cool completely in the pan before slicing.

10. Once cooled, cut the brownies into squares and serve.

Raspberry Coconut Bars:

- Preparation time: 15 minutes

- Cooking time: 25 minutes

- Chilling time: 2 hours

- Servings: 12 bars

Ingredients:

- 1 and 1/2 cups graham cracker crumbs

- 1/2 cup unsalted butter, melted

- 1 cup shredded coconut

- 1 can (14 ounces) sweetened condensed milk

- 1 cup fresh or frozen raspberries

Directions:

1. Preheat your oven to 350°F (175°C). Grease or line an 8x8-inch baking pan.

2. In a bowl, combine the graham cracker crumbs and melted butter. Mix until the crumbs are evenly coated.

3. Press the crumb mixture into the bottom of the prepared baking pan to form the crust.

4. Sprinkle the shredded coconut over the crust, creating an even layer.

5. Pour the sweetened condensed milk evenly over the coconut layer, making sure to cover the entire surface.

6. Scatter the raspberries over the condensed milk layer.

7. Bake in the preheated oven for 25 minutes or until the edges are golden brown and the center is set.

8. Remove from the oven and let the raspberry coconut bars cool in the pan for 10 minutes.

9. Transfer the bars to a wire rack and allow them to cool completely.

10. Once cooled, refrigerate the bars for at least 2 hours to firm up.

11. Cut into bars and serve.

Peanut Butter Chocolate Chip Cookies:

- Preparation time: 15 minutes

- Cooking time: 10-12 minutes

- Servings: Approximately 24 cookies

Ingredients:

- 1/2 cup unsalted butter, softened

- 1/2 cup peanut butter (smooth or chunky)

- 1/2 cup granulated sugar

- 1/2 cup packed brown sugar

- 1 large egg

- 1 teaspoon vanilla extract

- 1 and 1/4 cups all-purpose flour

- 1/2 teaspoon baking soda

- 1/4 teaspoon salt

- 1 cup chocolate chips

Directions:

1. Preheat your oven to 375°F (190°C). Line a baking sheet with parchment paper.

2. In a large bowl, cream together the softened butter, peanut butter, granulated sugar, and brown sugar until light and fluffy.

3. Beat in the egg and vanilla extract until well combined.

4. In a separate bowl, whisk together the all-purpose flour, baking soda, and salt.

5. Gradually add the dry ingredients to the wet ingredients, mixing until just combined.

6. Stir in the chocolate chips, distributing them evenly throughout the dough.

7. Drop rounded tablespoons of dough onto the prepared baking sheet, spacing them about 2 inches apart.

8. Flatten each cookie slightly with a fork, making a crisscross pattern.

9. Bake in the preheated oven for 10-12 minutes or until the cookies are golden brown around the edges.

10. Remove from the oven and let the cookies cool on the baking sheet for a few minutes before transferring them to a wire rack to cool completely.

11. Once cooled, store the peanut butter chocolate chip cookies in an airtight container. Enjoy!

Vanilla Bean Coconut Ice Cream:

- Preparation time: 10 minutes

- Chilling time: 4 hours or overnight

- Freezing time: 30 minutes in an ice cream maker

- Servings: 4

Ingredients:

- 2 cans (13.5 oz each) full-fat coconut milk

- 1/2 cup granulated sugar or sweetener of choice

- 1 vanilla bean, split lengthwise and seeds scraped out (or 1 teaspoon vanilla extract)

- Pinch of salt

Directions:

1. In a saucepan, combine the coconut milk, sugar, vanilla bean seeds (or vanilla extract), and salt. Heat the mixture over medium heat, stirring occasionally, until it begins to steam. Do not let it boil.

2. Remove the saucepan from the heat and let the mixture cool slightly.

3. Remove the vanilla bean pod (if using) and transfer the mixture to a container with a lid. Refrigerate for at least 4 hours or overnight to chill thoroughly.

4. Once chilled, pour the mixture into an ice cream maker and churn according to the manufacturer's instructions, usually around 30 minutes or until the ice cream reaches a soft-serve consistency.

5. Transfer the churned ice cream to a lidded container and freeze for an additional 2-4 hours, or until firm.

6. Serve the vanilla bean coconut ice cream in bowls or cones and enjoy its creamy, tropical flavor.

Lemon Berry Parfait:

- Preparation time: 10 minutes

- Servings: 2

Ingredients:

- 1 cup plain Greek yogurt

- 2 tablespoons honey or maple syrup

- Zest of 1 lemon

- 1 cup mixed berries (such as strawberries, blueberries, and raspberries)

- 1/4 cup granola

Directions:

1. In a bowl, mix together the Greek yogurt, honey or maple syrup, and lemon zest until well combined.

2. In serving glasses or bowls, layer the yogurt mixture, mixed berries, and granola.

3. Repeat the layers until all the ingredients are used, finishing with a dollop of yogurt and a sprinkle of granola on top.

4. Serve immediately or refrigerate until ready to serve.

5. Enjoy this refreshing and nutritious lemon berry parfait as a light breakfast or dessert.

Chocolate Chip Zucchini Bread:

- Preparation time: 15 minutes

- Baking time: 50-60 minutes

- Servings: 1 loaf

Ingredients:

- 1 and 1/2 cups all-purpose flour

- 1/2 cup cocoa powder

- 1 teaspoon baking soda

- 1/2 teaspoon baking powder

- 1/2 teaspoon salt

- 1/2 teaspoon ground cinnamon

- 1/2 cup unsalted butter, melted

- 1 cup granulated sugar

- 2 large eggs

- 1 teaspoon vanilla extract

- 1 and 1/2 cups shredded zucchini (about 1 medium zucchini)

- 1 cup chocolate chips

Directions:

1. Preheat your oven to 350°F (175°C). Grease a 9x5-inch loaf pan or line it with parchment paper.

2. In a bowl, whisk together the all-purpose flour, cocoa powder, baking soda, baking powder, salt, and ground cinnamon.

3. In a separate large bowl, cream together the melted butter and granulated sugar until well combined.

4. Add the eggs, one at a time, beating well after each addition. Stir in the vanilla extract.

5. Gradually add the dry ingredients to the wet ingredients, mixing until just combined.

6. Fold in the shredded zucchini and chocolate chips, ensuring they are evenly distributed throughout the batter.

7. Pour the batter into the prepared loaf pan, smoothing the top with a spatula.

8. Bake in the preheated oven for 50-60 minutes or until a toothpick inserted into the center comes out clean or with a few moist crumbs.

9. Remove from the oven and let the zucchini bread cool in the pan for 10 minutes before transferring it to a wire rack to cool completely.

10. Once cooled, slice the chocolate chip zucchini bread and enjoy it as a delicious snack or dessert.

Caramelized Banana Sundaes:

- Preparation time: 5 minutes

- Cooking time: 5 minutes

- Servings: 2

Ingredients:

- 2 ripe bananas, peeled and sliced

- 2 tablespoons unsalted butter

- 2 tablespoons brown sugar

- 2 tablespoons chopped nuts (such as walnuts or pecans)

- Vanilla ice cream or frozen yogurt

- Optional toppings: chocolate sauce, whipped cream, maraschino cherries

Directions:

1. In a non-stick skillet, melt the butter over medium heat.

2. Add the sliced bananas to the skillet and sprinkle them with brown sugar.

3. Cook the bananas for about 2-3minutes on each side, until they are golden and caramelized.

4. Remove the skillet from the heat and let the caramelized bananas cool slightly.

5. Scoop vanilla ice cream or frozen yogurt into serving bowls or glasses.

6. Top the ice cream with the caramelized bananas, sprinkle with chopped nuts, and drizzle with any optional toppings you desire, such as chocolate sauce or whipped cream.

7. Serve the caramelized banana sundaes immediately and enjoy the warm, sweet flavors combined with cool and creamy ice cream.

Mixed Berry Frozen Yogurt:

- Preparation time: 5 minutes

- Freezing time: 4-6 hours

- Servings: 4

Ingredients:

- 3 cups mixed berries (such as strawberries, blueberries, and raspberries), fresh or frozen

- 2 cups plain Greek yogurt

- 1/4 cup honey or maple syrup (adjust according to sweetness preference)

- 1 teaspoon vanilla extract

Directions:

1. If using frozen berries, let them thaw slightly at room temperature for about 10 minutes.

2. In a blender or food processor, combine the mixed berries, Greek yogurt, honey or maple syrup, and vanilla extract.

3. Blend the mixture until smooth and well combined.

4. Pour the mixture into an ice cream maker and churn according to the manufacturer's instructions, usually around 20-30 minutes or until the frozen yogurt reaches a soft-serve consistency.

5. Transfer the churned frozen yogurt to a lidded container and freeze for an additional 4-6 hours, or until firm.

6. Before serving, let the frozen yogurt sit at room temperature for a few minutes to soften slightly.

7. Scoop the mixed berry frozen yogurt into bowls or cones and enjoy its refreshing and fruity taste.

Chapter 7:

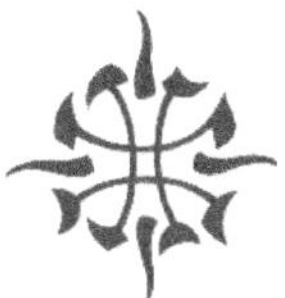

CONCLUSION AND FINAL THOUGHTS

Celebrating your journey with the SIBO Biphasic diet:

Congratulations on completing your journey with the SIBO Biphasic diet! It's a significant achievement and a testament to your dedication and commitment to improving your health. This diet plays a crucial role in managing small intestinal bacterial overgrowth (SIBO) and restoring balance to your gut.

Reflecting on the benefits and challenges of the diet:

As you look back on your experience with the SIBO Biphasic diet, take a moment to acknowledge the positive impacts it has had on your health. This diet aims to reduce the overgrowth of bacteria in the small intestine and alleviate symptoms such as bloating, gas, and digestive discomfort. By following the diet's guidelines, you may have experienced relief from these symptoms and noticed an improvement in your overall well-being.

However, it's important to acknowledge the challenges you faced throughout this journey. Adhering to a restrictive diet can be difficult, and you may have encountered moments of frustration or temptation. Remember that these challenges are normal and part of the process. Your determination and perseverance have brought you to this point, and that's worth celebrating.

Maintaining a healthy lifestyle beyond the SIBO Biphasic diet:

Now that you have completed the SIBO Biphasic diet, it's essential to transition into a sustainable and healthy lifestyle. While the diet may have provided temporary relief, it's important to continue implementing habits that support your gut health and overall well-being.

Consider incorporating the following practices into your daily routine:

- Focus on a well-balanced diet that includes a variety of nutrient-dense foods, such as fruits, vegetables, lean proteins, whole grains, and healthy fats.

- Stay hydrated by drinking an adequate amount of water throughout the day.

- Prioritize stress management techniques, such as meditation, yoga, or engaging in activities you enjoy.

- Establish a regular exercise routine that suits your preferences and physical abilities.

- Get sufficient sleep to support your body's healing and recovery processes.

- Consult with a healthcare professional or registered dietitian to develop a personalized plan that aligns with your specific needs and health goals.

Encouragement and support for continued success:

As you continue on your journey towards optimal health, remember that success is not always linear. There may be ups and downs along the way, but every step forward counts. Embrace the progress you have made and stay motivated to maintain a healthy lifestyle.

Surround yourself with a support system that understands and encourages your goals. Share your experiences with loved ones, join support groups, or seek guidance from healthcare professionals who specialize in gut health. Building a network of support can provide you with valuable insights, advice, and encouragement when you need it most.

Acknowledgments and gratitude:

Take a moment to express gratitude for yourself and those who have supported you throughout your journey. Recognize your own strength, resilience, and commitment to improving your health. Also, express appreciation for the individuals who have been there for you every step of the way—family, friends, healthcare professionals, and anyone who has provided guidance and support.

Remember that you are not alone on this journey, and there are resources and communities available to help you. Celebrate your achievements, learn from the challenges, and continue moving forward with confidence and determination. Wishing you continued success and a healthy, vibrant life ahead.